Advances in Forefoot Surgery

Editor

CHARLES M. ZELEN

CLINICS IN PODIATRIC MEDICINE AND SURGERY

www.podiatric.theclinics.com

Consulting Editor
THOMAS ZGONIS

July 2013 • Volume 30 • Number 3

ELSEVIER

1600 John F. Kennedy Boulevard • Suite 1800 • Philadelphia, Pennsylvania, 19103-2899

http://www.theclinics.com

CLINICS IN PODIATRIC MEDICINE AND SURGERY Volume 30, Number 3
July 2013 ISSN 0891-8422, ISBN-13: 978-1-4557-7608-5

Editor: Patrick Manley

Clinics in Podiatric Medicine and Surgery (ISSN 0891-8422) is published quarterly by Elsevier Inc., 360 Park Avenue South, New York, NY 10010-1710. Months of issue are January, April, July, and October. Business and Editorial Offices: 1600 John F. Kennedy Blvd., Ste. 1800, Philadelphia, PA 19103-2899. Customer Service Office: 3251 Riverport Lane, Maryland Heights, MO 63043. Periodicals postage paid at New York, NY and additional mailing offices. Subscription prices are $292.00 per year for US individuals, $410.00 per year for US institutions, $148.00 per year for US students and residents, $350.00 per year for Canadian individuals, $508.00 for Canadian institutions, $415.00 for international individuals, $508.00 per year for international institutions and $208.00 per year for Canadian and foreign students/residents. To receive student/resident rate, orders must be accompanied by name of affiliated institution, date of term, and the *signature* of program/residency coordinator on institution letterhead. Orders will be billed at individual rate until proof of status is received. Foreign air speed delivery is included in all *Clinics* subscription prices. All prices are subject to change without notice. POSTMASTER: Send address changes to *Clinics in Podiatric Medicine and Surgery*, Elsevier Health Sciences Division, Subscription Customer Service, 3251 Riverport Lane, Maryland Heights, MO 63043. **Customer Service: 1-800-654-2452 (US). From outside of the US, call 314-447-8871. Fax: 314-447-8029. E-mail: JournalsCustomerService-usa@elsevier.com (for print support); JournalsOnlineSupport-usa@elsevier.com (for online support).**

Reprints. For copies of 100 or more of articles in this publication, please contact the Commercial Reprints Department, Elsevier Inc., 360 Park Avenue South, New York, NY 10010-1710. Tel.: 212-633-3812; Fax: 212-462-1935; E-mail: reprints@elsevier.com.

Clinics in Podiatric Medicine and Surgery is covered in *MEDLINE/PubMed (Index Medicus) and EMBASE/Excerpta Medica.*

Printed and bound by CPI Group (UK) Ltd, Croydon, CR0 4YY

Transferred to digital print 2013

CLINICS IN PODIATRIC MEDICINE AND SURGERY

Contributors

CONSULTING EDITOR

THOMAS ZGONIS, DPM, FACFAS
Associate Professor, Externship and Fellowship Director in Reconstructive Foot and Ankle Surgery, Division of Podiatric Medicine and Surgery, Department of Orthopaedic Surgery, University of Texas Health Science Center at San Antonio, San Antonio, Texas

EDITOR

CHARLES M. ZELEN, DPM, FACFAS, FACFAOM
Foot and Ankle Associates of Southwest Virginia, Salem, Virginia; Director, Professional Education and Research Institute, Roanoke, Virginia

AUTHORS

ERIGENA BAZE, DPM
Resident, Heritage Valley Hospital Beaver, Beaver, Pennsylvania

DREW CHRISTIE, DPM
Resident, Foot and Ankle Residency Program, Saint Vincent's Hospital, Indianapolis, Indiana

J. RANDOLPH CLEMENTS, DPM
Assistant Professor, Surgery, Virgina Tech Carilion School of Medicine, Carilion Clinic Orthopedics, Roanoke, Virginia

LESTER DENNIS, DPM, FACFAS
Attending Surgeon, Division of Podiatric Surgery, Department of Surgery, Wyckoff Heights Medical Center, Brooklyn, New York

LAWRENCE DIDOMENICO, DPM
Director of Fellowship Training, Adjunct Professor; Ankle and Foot Care Centers/Kent State University College of Podiatric Medicine, Youngstown, Ohio; Saint Elizabeth Medical Center, Youngstown, Ohio

NIKOLAY GATALYAK, DPM
Private Practice Ankle and Foot Care Centers, Columbiana, Ohio

KELLIE HIGGINS, DPM
Resident, Foot and Ankle Residency Program, Saint Vincent's Hospital, Indianapolis, Indiana

TAHIR KHAN, DPM
Second Year Resident, Division of Podiatric Surgery, Department of Surgery, Wyckoff Heights Medical Center, Brooklyn, New York

DAVID L. NIELSON, DPM, AACFAS
Foot and Ankle Associates of Southwest Virginia, Salem, Virginia

VICTOR NWOSU, DPM
Fellow, American Health Network Reconstructive Foot and Ankle Surgical Fellowship, Indianapolis, Indiana

ADAM D. PERLER, DPM, FACFAS
Chief of Podiatric Surgery, Saint Vincent's Hospital System; Attending, American Health Network Reconstructive Foot and Ankle Surgical Fellowship; Attending, Foot and Ankle Residency Program, Saint Vincent's Hospital, Indianapolis, Indiana

CHRISTOPHER REEVES, DPM, FACFAS
Orlando Foot and Ankle Clinics, Winter Park, Florida

ROBERT SCHOPF, DPM
PGY-1, Carilion Clinic Podiatric Medicine and Surgery, Roanoke, Virginia

AMBER SHANE, DPM, FACFAS
Orlando Foot and Ankle Clinics, Orlando, Florida

JASON SNYDER, DPM
Third Year Resident, Division of Podiatric Surgery, Department of Surgery, Wyckoff Heights Medical Center, Brooklyn, New York

BRIAN S. STOVER, DPM
Southeastern Sports Medicine, Asheville, North Carolina

PAUL THURSTON, DPM
Chief Resident, PGY-3, Florida Hospital East Orlando, Orlando, Florida

JOSEPH R. TREADWELL, DPM
Private Practice, Foot and Ankle Specialists of CT, Danbury, Connecticut

GARRETT WOBST, DPM
Chief Resident, PGY-3, Florida Hospital East Orlando, Orlando, Florida

NATHAN J. YOUNG, DPM, AACFAS, AAFAS
Foot and Ankle Associates of Southwest Virginia, Salem, Virginia; Surgical and Research Fellow, Professional Education and Research Institute, Roanoke, Virginia

CHARLES M. ZELEN, DPM, FACFAS, FACFAOM
Foot and Ankle Associates of Southwest Virginia, Salem, Virginia; Medical Director, Professional Education and Research Institute, Roanoke, Virginia

Contents

> For lesser toe deformities, fusion of the proximal interphalangeal joint offers good long-term correction and predictability. Digital arthrodesis has been described for longer than 100 years in the literature, and current techniques closely resemble those described in early accounts. However, many implants currently being used take advantage of the latest metallurgic and polymeric innovations, with implants being composed of nitinol, polylactic or polyglycolic acids, and polydioxanone. Newer implants offer easy insertion and good stability, with no percutaneous wires. Pin-tract infection rates from exposed Kirschner wires may be as high as 18%, and newer implants help to mitigate this problem.

> After 4 to 8 weeks of normal primary bone healing, rigid internal fixation is no longer required. Newer generation absorbable implants have become reliable and cost-effective alternatives to metallic hardware. Modern implants are formulated to have increased strength and smoother resorption over the course of 18 to 24 months, which decreases the possibility of local inflammation. Historically, bioresorbable screws can be time consuming to insert, but newer devices are being developed that help ease their insertion. A case of a bunionectomy is presented with double osteotomy on a 40-year-old nurse fixated with polyglycolic acid and poly-L-lactic acid copolymer screws.

> The surgical correction of hallux valgus has evolved since it was first described. Many osteotomies and fixation methods have been described and results have improved. Innovative new fixation methods include the Mini TightRope, new absorbable implants, and plating options. This article discusses the evolution of capital osteotomies as well as the evolution of fixation. Also presented is a case study of a novel method of achieving solid fixation across an osteotomy using a high-frequency sonic device to insert a bioresorbable pin.

> Correction of the fifth digit deformity and Tailor's Bunion can be rewarding as well as challenging for a foot and ankle surgeon. Immense care should be taken when performing these reconstructive surgical procedure, especially to avoid and minimize complication rates and mainly to prevent neurovascular damage. Appropriate surgical procedure selection for the fifth digit deformity and Tailor's Bunion is necessary in order to obtain a long term predictable outcome.

> Arthrodesis of the first metatarsocuneiform joint is a powerful and durable procedure to help correct moderate to severe hallux valgus and/or first ray hypermobility. However, painful nonunion remains a notoriously high potential outcome. Research regarding locking plates seems promising, and data show lower rates of nonunion. Innovative fixation techniques are new and should be considered in the future as further literature is available on their long-term use. Regardless of the fixation, proper joint preparation and good compression is fundamentally the most important. A case of Lapidus fusion with locking plates after a failed arthrodesis with screws alone is presented.

> Forefoot traumas, particularly involving the metatarsals, are commonly occurring injuries. There have been several advances in management of these injuries. These advances include updates in operative technique, internal fixation options, plating constructs, and external fixation. In addition, the advances of soft tissue management have improved outcomes. This article outlines these injuries and provides an update on techniques, principles, and understanding of managing forefoot trauma.

Current Concepts and Techniques in Foot and Ankle Surgery

> A retrospective review of 7 patients (8 total feet) was conducted by the authors to determine the effects of combined 1st metatarsal Reverdin-Laird and opening base wedge osteotomy in the management of hallux valgus deformity. Postoperative radiographs were compared with preoperative radiographs for improvement in the 1st intermetatarsal angle, proximal articular set angle, hallux abductus angle, and tibial sesamoid position.

Advances in Forefoot Surgery

CLINICS IN PODIATRIC MEDICINE AND SURGERY

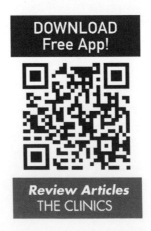

Foreword

Forefoot Surgery

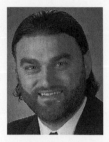

Thomas Zgonis, DPM, FACFAS
Consulting Editor

This edition of *Clinics in Podiatric Medicine and Surgery* is focused on the indications and contraindications of forefoot surgical reconstruction including and not limited to hallux abducto valgus and hallux rigidus repair, digital deformity correction, and second metatarsophalangeal joint pathology. Various first metatarsal osteotomies and first metatarsocuneiform arthrodesis procedures are described in detail for the correction of symptomatic hallux abducto valgus deformities. Equal attention is emphasized for the correction of digital deformities, Tailor's bunion, and management of forefoot trauma. Last, alternative methods of absorbable fixation in forefoot surgery are also discussed in detail.

Forefoot pathology is very common and surgical reconstruction can become quite challenging when dealing with biomechanical abnormalities, neuromuscular disorders, and revisional surgery. In this issue, the guest editor, Dr Zelen, along with the invited authors have done an excellent job in addressing some of the most common deformities in the forefoot that can be used as a great reference to our readers. I thank you again for your outstanding submissions.

Thomas Zgonis, DPM, FACFAS
Division of Podiatric Medicine and Surgery
Department of Orthopaedic Surgery
University of Texas Health Science Center at San Antonio
7703 Floyd Curl Drive–MSC 7776
San Antonio, TX 78229, USA

E-mail address:
zgonis@uthscsa.edu

Clin Podiatr Med Surg 30 (2013) xi
http://dx.doi.org/10.1016/j.cpm.2013.05.001
0891-8422/13/$ – see front matter © 2013 Published by Elsevier Inc.

podiatric.theclinics.com

Preface

Advances in Forefoot Surgery

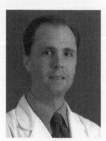

Charles M. Zelen, DPM, FACFAS, FACFAOM
Editor

Reconstructive surgery to the forefoot is the most common and in many instances the most challenging pathologic abnormality the foot and ankle surgeon undertakes in the operative suite. Obtaining excellent and reproducible results over the long term in our patients is a common goal we stride for in our careers.

While the procedures we perform in the forefoot remain similar over the years, the techniques and hardware made available to us have evolved. Many of the changes brought improvements to our surgical outcomes. Advances in biologic products, screws, locking plates, and anatomic specific hardware paved the way to these successes.

In this issue of *Clinics in Podiatric Medicine and Surgery*, I was given the opportunity to select several unique advances that span from digital surgery, to the first ray, to lesser metatarsals and tailor's bunions, as well as to trauma applications. I am privileged to have such an experienced and dynamic group of authors contribute to this edition.

I would like each of the readers to take a moment and consider what techniques and fixation modalities you are currently using. Ponder the possibility of modifying and adapting to some of what the authors present in this edition into your own practice. You will have the opportunity to review and analyze many of the advanced techniques, applications, and alternatives in hardware in this edition. Each article is innovative and will allow you to consider other alternatives in your practice. However, it is always necessary and imperative to ask the questions, what is too complex and when are we going "overboard"?

We begin with digital arthrodesis, and the complexity of the hammertoe deformity with a brief review of the new implants available. Resorbable fixation, an ongoing controversy in forefoot surgery, is also reviewed. Different options for fixation of capital osteotomies as well as a unique method for chevron fixation are introduced. Newer advances in base wedge procedures, second metatarsal phalangeal joint pathologic

Clin Podiatr Med Surg 30 (2013) xiii–xiv
http://dx.doi.org/10.1016/j.cpm.2013.05.002
0891-8422/13/$ – see front matter © 2013 Published by Elsevier Inc.

condition, and tailor's bunion procedures are analyzed as well. We then delve into the complexity of the first metatarsal phalangeal joint arthroplasty and fusion, where there are many new developments that have come to light over the past decade. Lapidus and the anatomic plating available are discussed in depth and a brief review of advances in trauma surgery of the forefoot rounds out our edition.

While it seems that the number, variety, and often complexity of forefoot implants grow considerably each year, the truth is we only scratched the surface. I foresee many more product advances that are still in the developmental phase, including the possibility of antibiotic-coated hardware, resorbable screws mixed with antibiotics, as well as bone glues and screws that stimulate bone formation. This is only a short list in product advancement that the future may hold. Over the last decade, many foot and ankle surgeons marvel at the advances in forefoot surgery. My friends, I ask that you please stay tuned; there is still much to look forward to.

Respectfully submitted for your continued education.

Charles M. Zelen, DPM, FACFAS, FACFAOM
Foot and Ankle Associates of Southwest Virginia
1802 Braeburn Drive, Ste M120
Salem, VA 24153, USA

Professional Education and Research Institute
222 Walnut Avenue
Roanoke, VA 24016, USA

E-mail address:
cmzelen@periedu.com

Digital Arthrodesis

Charles M. Zelen, DPM, FACFAS, FACFAOM[a,b,]*,
Nathan J. Young, DPM, AACFAS, AAFAS[a,b]

KEYWORDS

- Hammer toe • Arthrodesis • StayFuse • SmartToe • ProToe

KEY POINTS

- Lesser toe deformities are a common complaint encountered by the foot and ankle surgeon.
- Arthrodesis is indicated when there is a recurrence or rigidity of the deformity and when conservative treatment has failed. Arthrodesis offers a high degree of predictability, with the only disadvantage being an inability of the toe to bend at the center joint.
- Kirschner wires are frequently used to stabilize the osteotomy, but are associated with complications such as pin-tract infections, nonunion or malunion from achieving stability in only one plane and wire loosening, patient anxiety from the exposed wires, and pain associated with removal of the wire or bumping the wire end while ambulating. Newer implants seek to eliminate these difficulties by offering enhanced stability and compression, simple insertion, and no exposed hardware.

INTRODUCTION

Deformities of the lesser digits, such as hammer toes, claw toes, and mallet toes, are among the most frequent patient complaints encountered by foot surgeons. There are multiple causes for these deformities, with the underlying pathology arising from flexor stabilization, flexor substitution, or extensor substitution in most instances. Irrespective of the etiology, there are common anatomic considerations that tend to guide the treatment in clinical practice.[1]

Arthroplasty or arthrodesis of the interphalangeal joint is most commonly used to help correct the deformities. These procedures are frequently performed with other adjunctive procedures such as digital tendon transfers, metatarsophalangeal (MTP) joint releases, and metatarsal osteotomies to correct the more pervasive forefoot deformities.

Soule[2] first described fusion of a lesser interphalangeal joint in 1910. He described a plantar approach and postoperative plaster splintage. The procedure has since been modified by the peg-in-hole configuration,[3,4] Kirschner-wire fixation,[5] AO screws and

[a] Foot and Ankle Associates of Southwest Virginia, 1802 Braeburn Drive, Suite M120, Salem, VA 24153, USA; [b] Professional Education and Research Institute, 222 Walnut Avenue, Roanoke, VA 24016, USA
* Corresponding author.
E-mail address: cmzelen@periedu.com

Clin Podiatr Med Surg 30 (2013) 271–282
http://dx.doi.org/10.1016/j.cpm.2013.04.006
0891-8422/13/$ – see front matter © 2013 Published by Elsevier Inc.

staples, and, more recently, newer metallic and absorbable devices designed specifically for interphalangeal fusion of lesser digits. Newer devices combine ease of use with reliable fixation and fusion.

Digital deformities have been found to be more common in persons of African American descent than in Caucasians, and afflict females more commonly than males. Advancing age also correlates with increasing incidence.[6] Many factors may predispose patients to digital contracture, such as pes cavus, pes planus, ankle equinus, abnormal metatarsal parabola, neuromuscular conditions, arthritides, trauma, adjacent digit-deforming forces (ie, hallux valgus), or improperly fitted shoes and/or hosiery.[1,6,7]

Hammer-toe syndrome is a term that describes multiple symptoms and joint disturbances affecting the MTP and interphalangeal joints. These deformities include hammer toes (plantarflexion at the proximal interphalangeal [PIP] joint), claw toes (plantarflexion at both the PIP and the distal interphalangeal [DIP] joints), mallet toes (plantarflexion at the DIP joint), overlapping fifth toe, and clinodactyly or curly toe. With the exception of clinodactyly, the contractures are generally acquired deformities[6] that typically result from an imbalance of the long flexors and extensors, which overpowers the intrinsic and/or extrinsic muscles of the digits and their associated MTP joints.[1] This musculoskeletal imbalance may arise from many possible origins including flexor stabilization, extensor substitution, or extensor stabilization.

Instability of the MTP joints from age-related changes or gait, as well as inflammatory conditions such as rheumatoid arthritis, can lead to contracture of the digits. In addition, neuromuscular conditions, such as Charcot-Marie-Tooth disease, may lead to digital deformities. When multiple claw toes are present, an underlying neurologic condition should be considered.[8]

Clinically the patient may have varied symptomatology. Patients may exhibit hyperkeratotic clavi, ulceration, and/or adventitious bursae, which may or may not be painful, erythematous, or infected. The digits should be assessed as to whether the deformities are flexible or rigid. The contractures should be assessed in non–weight-bearing as well as weight-bearing positions.

Before surgical intervention it is recommended that conservative treatment measures be exhausted. These treatments might include orthoses, toe splints and padding, shoe modifications, keratolytics, debridement of painful lesions, and anti-inflammatories (injections or oral medication). Some patients receive adequate benefit from conservative treatment initially, although many may require surgical intervention at a later time.

Surgical corrections of lesser toe deformities are some of the most frequently performed procedures on the forefoot.[9] Surgical treatment options include tenotomy/capsulotomy, arthroplasty, arthrodesis, and tendon-balancing procedures. Arthrodesis is the most common procedure performed and is indicated in the following instances: recurrent and/or progressive flexible deformity, neuromuscular deformity, transverse plane deformity, and semirigid and rigid deformity[10,11] There is a multitude of techniques such as peg-in-hole fusion, chevron osteotomy of the joint,[12] conical reaming of the joint,[13] or end-to-end fusion. In addition, a multitude of devices is available for the treatment of lesser digit deformities, including both absorbable and metallic devices. Some devices such as cerclage wire, AO screws, staples, Kirschner wires, and absorbable pins are nonspecific for hammer-toe correction but are used nonetheless. Other devices such as the Weil-Carver Hammer Toe Implant (Biomet, Warsaw, IN), Pro-Toe (Wright Medical Technology, Arlington, TN), StayFuse (Tornier, Edina, MN), and SmartToe (Stryker, Mahwah NJ), which are intended only for hammer-toe fusion, have become more popular of late.

Peg-in-hole fixation methods have long been advocated for fixation of digital arthrodeses. The technique can be stabilized by impaction of the medullary bone, with a Kirschner wire used for added stability. The peg-in-hole technique does provide good stability, but is technically more demanding to perform and can provide significant shortening of the digit.[3,4,14] Other choices such as conical reaming and chevron osteotomies are less commonly used in most clinical practices. The most popular choice with surgeons is still the end-to-end technique for fusion, with Kirschner wires serving as the most widely used choice for fixation.

Resorbable implants for fixation have a place in hammer-toe correction and have been used for many years. Early-generation resorbable devices provided adequate rigidity for bone healing, but were resorbed so quickly that they would predispose the tissue to an inflammatory reaction. Over the last 15 years the resorbable implants have been reformulated without dyes, with a lower content of polyglycolic acid and a higher content of polylactic acid. These changes have dramatically decreased the inflammatory reactions that were common in earlier devices.[15] Blending the polymers in various compositions causes the implant to have a more favorable strength and absorption profile.[16] Common resorbable devices used in lesser digit arthrodeses include pins that can be smooth, tapered, or textured.

Numerous orthopedic device companies make resorbable pins including the RFS pin (Tornier, Edina, MN), ReUnite (BioMet, Warsaw, IN), TrimIt and Bio-Compression Pins (Arthrex, Naples, FL), and SmartPin (ConMed Linvatec, Largo, FL), to name a few. Each pin has a unique formulation that dictates the device's strength and resorption characteristics. In most instances these resorbable pins are easy to insert, eliminate the risk of pin-tract infections, do not protrude from the skin, and do not require removal. Absorbable pins do not provide much compression, if any. Patient perception, however, is very favorable, as there is no metallic implant remaining in the toes, and the implant will dissolve slowly over time. In addition, because the pins are resorbed through hydrolysis, they are considered bacteriostatic in nature and there is a lower risk of infection.

One unique resorbable device is the Weil-Carver hammer-toe implant, which is in the shape of a screw/barbed pin specifically designed for digital arthrodeses. This device is partially threaded on the proximal end and is barbed on the distal end, providing a press fit. This shape helps to achieve good stability and a small amount of compression, and prevents pistoning across the toe fusion.[17]

Another truly resorbable implant that is used for hammer-toe fusion is the cadaveric bone dowel. Allogenic bone implants have been used since the advent of bone banking in the 1940s. Dowels can be formed from the freeze-dried allograft and inserted across an osteotomy. Unlike metallic implants and other resorbable implants, cortical bone pins provide an osteoconductive substrate and are replaced via creeping substitution.[18] Creeping substitution is the process by which bone is resorbed via osteoclastic action and new vascular channels, and bone is formed via osteoblastic action, resulting in new Haversian canal systems.[19] Cortical bone pins have low tissue reactivity and adequate strength, but provide minimal compression and present a small risk of disease transmission.

Metallic hardware still remains the more popular choice for fixation because of its high strength, versatility, ease of insertion, and low tissue reactivity. However, metallic implants are considerably stiffer than bone, which can cause osteopenia owing to stress shielding, and a second surgery may be required for hardware removal. Common metals used in orthopedic implants include surgical stainless steel and titanium alloys.

Stainless steel has long been used as an implant in orthopedic surgery because it is strong, relatively cheap, and easy to manufacture. However, it does possess poor wear attributes as a force-bearing surface as well as a poor corrosion profile. Therefore, aside from standard screws and wire fixation, the majority of specialty implants for hammer toes are made from titanium alloys.

Titanium alloys composed of titanium, aluminum, and vanadium are extremely inert and are resistant to corrosion.[20] Such titanium alloys have low moduli of elasticity and low tensile strengths, therefore these implants need to be bulkier than implants made of stainless steel. A newer titanium alloy used in orthopedic implants is nickel-titanium, or nitinol. This innovative metal has a unique ability to remember its original shape after being deformed by increasing its temperature.[21] This change in shape can provide compression across an osteotomy or fusion site.

In addition to the standard Kirschner wire, stainless-steel wires can be used to provide stabilization across toe-fusion sites.[22] Stainless-steel wires range in size, but 20- or 22-gauge wire provides a good balance between stiffness and strength. Holes are drilled on either side of the osteotomy, after which the wire is passed through and tightened. This form of fixation is relatively simple and requires minimal instrumentation. It has also been shown to be highly resistant to displacement.[23] The disadvantage of this method of fixation is that the wire can pull through the cortical bone, and thus requires good bone density for success.

As mentioned earlier, the Kirschner wire remains the most popular form of fixation for hammer toes. Taylor[5] first used Kirschner wires to stabilize a digital arthrodesis in 1940. This modification allowed for more reliable fusion in digital deformities. Overall, Kirschner wires are easy to implant and explant, and are inexpensive. The downside, however, is that they can migrate and provide stability in only one plane. Patient satisfaction has always been an issue with this method of fixation, as patients may be concerned about having a pin sticking out of their toe, and the exposed wire can get caught on dressings, clothing, and furniture, causing pain and anxiety as well as unwanted retraction or breakage of the device. Pin-tract infections can also be a concern, such infections ranging between 1.8% and 18% in the literature.[24,25]

A less common form of hammer-toe fixation is the cannulated compression screw. This form of fixation provides the most interfragmentary compression across the fusion site among all fixation options. Using cannulated screws does sacrifice the DIP joint to fuse the PIP joint, but it can also minimize any subsequent angular deformities as a result.[26] Another potential disadvantage is that the patient may have persistent pain on the distal aspect of the toe that may require hardware removal. One distinct advantage is the usefulness of the cannulation in the screw so that if the MTP joint requires further stabilization after the correction of the toe deformity, a Kirschner wire can be left in place to cross the MTP joint.[27]

The Stayfuse hammer-toe implant (Tornier) is a 2-component titanium alloy device used for digital arthrodeses. The design allows for relatively easy insertion.[17] Before surgery, templates are used to determine the size of the patient's implants based on the preoperative radiographs. The medullary canals are prepared using a drill, and each component is then screwed into the bone. The proximal end is the female receptacle and the distal component has the male prong.[28] The device is press-fitted together to engage the two sides, making audible clicks as it engages. There is no percutaneous hardware, and the device, once fully engaged, provides good strength and stability. It may be difficult to correctly seat the device if the osteotomy is not completely parallel or if there is any soft tissue or boney tissue impinging on the osteotomy. A distinct advantage is the taper lock of the device, so that once the device is engaged it will not unsnap unless the surgeon uses a special tool (available in the kit). In addition, the implant provides good rotational stability and does not require entry into the MTP joint or DIP joint if it is not warranted.

ProToe VO is a single-component implant designed specifically for digital arthrodesis by Wright Medical. It is threaded on the proximal end and barbed on the distal end, very similar to the Weil-Carver resorbable device. The proximal end is screwed into place and the distal end is press-fitted into the middle phalanx.[29] The potential benefits include no percutaneous hardware, enhanced stability, and some compression. The device is also relatively easy to insert, and does not violate the distal or proximal joints.

Stryker Orthopedics has a unique intramedullary shape-memory nickel-titanium hammer-toe implant called the SmartToe. There are versions for both PIP joint and DIP joint available to meet surgeons' specific needs. After preparing the medullary canals with a drill and a brooch, the deformed device is implanted into the bone. Once the device is heated to the body's temperature it will retain its original shape and compress the two ends of the osteotomy.[30] The device is also available in various angles to give some plantarflexion if desired. This device is relatively easy to insert and is very reliable. However, it must be refrigerated before insertion, and can be very difficult to remove if it fails.[10]

SURGICAL TECHNIQUE

Surgery is recommended for patients who fail conservative treatments for their symptomatic digital deformities. Frequently patients who undergo lesser digit surgery also undergo other concurrent surgeries of the foot. It is important to diagnose and address other foot abnormalities that may also require surgical correction. When other procedures are performed, such as hallux valgus correction or metatarsal osteotomies, the digital arthrodeses are typically the last deformities corrected.

Once placed on the operating-room table in the supine position, a pneumatic ankle, calf, or thigh tourniquet is applied, depending on other concurrent procedures, if any, to provide hemostasis. Anesthesia may be obtained through typical means via digital, ankle, popliteal, spinal, or general anesthesia. Once sterilely prepped and draped, the surgeon's attention is directed to the digital deformity. In an isolated PIP joint fusion, a linear longitudinal incision or a transverse elliptical incision may be made over the joint. A transverse tenotomy is made through the extensor tendons to expose the joint. A #64 blade is used to perform a capsulotomy and cut the collateral ligaments, and further expose the head proximal phalanx. Once the soft tissue is retracted, the bones are then osteotomized.

The osteotomy can be performed in several ways. The bone can be cut in a peg-in-hole fashion, a chevron fashion, by conical reaming of the joint, or in end-to-end fashion. Each method presents benefits and shortcomings. The peg-in-hole and chevron osteotomies provide good bone-to-bone contact and stability, but may unacceptably shorten the digit. Conical reaming requires specialized instrumentation that may not be available. End-to-end fusion is simple to perform and provides minimal shortening, but is less stable and, if the osteotomies are not parallel, may provide an angular deformity of the digit. Given these potential advantages and disadvantages many surgeons prefer the end-to-end method, elaborated further here.

The head of the proximal phalanx can be osteotomized by use of a sagittal saw or bone-cutting forceps in an end-to-end fusion. This procedure is done with care to ensure good alignment in all planes to correct the preoperative deformity. Care is taken to excise only minimal bone to prevent postoperative shortening. In general, the proximal phalanx is resected within the flare of the neck and the middle phalanx is resected just enough to expose subchondral bone. At this time, the bone is prepared according to the fixation method of choice. After the procedure, the tendon is reapproximated, the skin is closed, and a dry, sterile dressing is applied to the foot.

Postoperative weight bearing depends on whether other concurrent procedures, if any, were performed. If only the digital arthrodesis was performed, in general partial weight bearing on the heel with the assistance of crutches will be allowed. Typically the patient is instructed to elevate the extremity and to use analgesics as required.

REHABILITATION AND RECOVERY

Typical recovery for hammer-toe surgery is relatively benign. Sutures are left in place for approximately 2 to 3 weeks and the patient may return to preoperative shoe gear once the swelling resolves and the wounds heal, if there are no other contraindications from so doing.

Complications may potentially include infection, prolonged swelling, recurrence or postsurgical deformity, or devascularization with possible loss of the toe. Fusion of the PIP joint can lead to symptomatic mallet toe in 8% to 44% of toes.[31] In rare instances postoperative vasoconstriction may complicate the healing process. Vasoconstriction can be seen after correction of a contracted digit that is subluxed or dislocated at the MTP joint. In such scenarios, the surgeon must ensure capillary filling in the operative suite. If the capillary refill is prolonged or the digit struggles to exhibit any reactive hyperemia, suture removal and/or fixation removal may be indicated. Doing this may decrease the surgical correction, but may prevent the loss of the digit. If the digit remains ischemic, it is vital to be proactive and to limit the amount of toe that is lost. Negative pressure devices and the application of topical nitroglycerin can help to increase local perfusion.

CASE STUDIES
Case Study #1

A 66-year-old healthy female science teacher presented to the clinic for evaluation of painful bunion and forefoot pain. She had tried and failed many conservative treatments for her pain including different shoes, orthotics, padding, and anti-inflammatories. On examination it was noted that she had a functional hallux limitus. She had pain with range of motion in the first MTP joint, and the total range of motion for the joint was decreased with a small dorsal ridge on the metatarsal. In addition, the hallux was impinging the second toe, owing to symptomatic pathologic hallux interphalangeus. She had pain on palpation of the second MTP joint that was prominent, and she had a rigidly contracted hammer toe on the second digit. She also had pain in the second intermetatarsal space. Her neurovascular status was intact. She did exhibit some erythema and edema on the affected digits.

A decompressional osteotomy of the first metatarsal and an Akin procedure were performed on the hallux with resorbable fixation, an osteotomy was performed on the second metatarsal, and the PIP joint was fused using a Stryker SmartToe implant (**Figs. 1** and **2**A, B).

Case Study #2

This patient was a 52-year-old woman who presented for evaluation of painful bunion and hammer toes. She is retired and is the primary caregiver to her husband, who is disabled. She had wanted to have surgery on her foot before this time, but was unable to do so owing to her caregiving responsibilities. Her foot was very painful and she also related burning in the second and third digits. On examination, it was revealed that she had a very significant bunion deformity with digits that were significantly contracted in the transverse and sagittal planes. The prominent joints were all painful to the touch. She had pain on palpation of the lesser second and third metatarsals. Radiographs

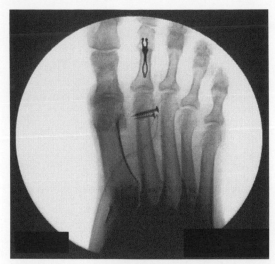

Fig. 1. Plain radiograph taken immediately after surgery. Note the SmartToe implant in the second digit with good correction and apposition.

revealed a very severe bunion deformity with significant subluxation of the first MTP joint. Dislocation of the second MTP joint was also evident (**Fig. 3**). It was decided that to reconstruct this patient's forefoot, a Lapidus procedure with Akin osteotomy would be performed in the hallux; arthrodeses would be performed in the second to fourth digits, and arthroplasty to the fifth; the second and third metatarsals would be osteotomized to shorten them; and a fifth metatarsal bunionectomy without osteotomy would be performed (**Fig. 4**). StayFuse implants were implanted into the PIP joints of the second to fourth digits, and an absorbable pin was inserted in the fifth digit to provide temporary fixation of that toe. All wounds and bone healed well. She has been followed up for more than 5 years and is very pleased with the overall outcome of the foot (**Fig. 5**).

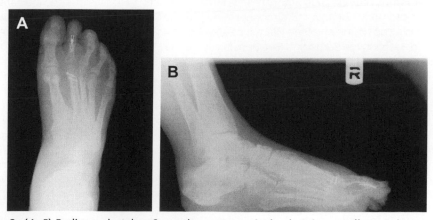

Fig. 2. (*A, B*) Radiographs taken 6 months postoperatively, showing excellent maintenance of correction. Note the curved nature of the SmartToe with the 10° plantar bend maintaining second-toe purchase.

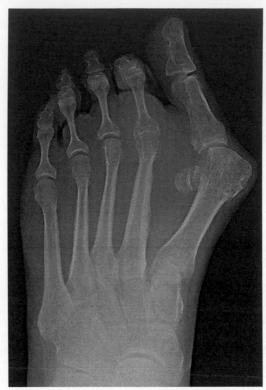

Fig. 3. Preoperative anteroposterior image. Note the very significant bunion deformity with hypertrophic metatarsal head, and the contracture of the second through fourth digits with the dorsal dislocation of the second digit at the MTP joint.

CLINICAL RESULTS IN THE LITERATURE

Nonunion rates of digital arthrodeses range between 0% and 35%.[32] However, fibrous ankylosis may provide satisfactory results in many patients.[14] Revision may be indicated in a symptomatic nonunion.[32] Kirschner wires provide stability in only one plane. Pseudarthrosis and nonunion of the PIP joint arthrodesis can cause residual toe pain and the need for revision toe surgery.[33] Pin-tract infections may be as high as 1.8% to 18%.[24,25] In an effort to minimize these risks, many new devices specifically designed for PIP joint fusion in symptomatic lesser toe deformities have been developed. Nonunion rates have been much lower with implantation of the newer orthopedic devices.

Ford and colleagues[18] performed digital arthrodeses on 30 toes with a cortical bone pin, and found 100% bony fusion and uneventful healing. Miller[34] performed PIP joint arthrodeses on 26 toes and found fusion in 25 of 26 toes. Fracture of the bone pin was found in 2 cases, 1 of which went on to symptomatic nonunion requiring revision surgery. This method may expose the patient to possible risk of disease transmission, albeit a very small one. All cadaveric bone was screened for human immunodeficiency virus and hepatitis B and C viruses, which were found in fewer than 6.3×10^{-7} samples.

Konkel and colleagues[35] corrected 48 lesser toe deformities using an absorbable pin. There was a 73% fusion rate in 48 toes with an additional 18% fibrous union. Also noted were 9 floating toes (18.8%) and postsurgical transverse plane deformity

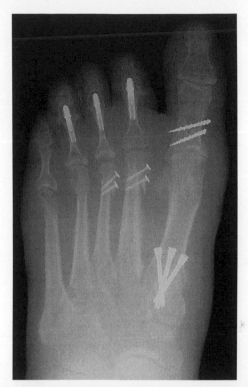

Fig. 4. Radiograph taken 3 months postoperatively. Note the good alignment of all digits.

in 8 toes (16.7%). Despite this, 91% of patients stated that they would have the surgery again. In another study in 47 toes with a newer bioabsorbable implant, Konkel and colleagues[31] reported 83% bony union. There was an increased number of floating toes (34%), but all but 2 of these toes had a concomitant Weil osteotomy performed. Ninety-three percent of patients reported that they would undergo the procedure again. In each of these 2 studies a few of the patients had previously undergone hammer-toe surgery on other digits, and greatly preferred the implanted device with no exposed hardware.

Cannulated screws for fusion of the PIP joint may provide significant ease of insertion, as this requires only one extra step beyond that of regular Kirschner-wire fixation. Lane[27] performed 20 fusions using a cannulated screw and noted that all went on to heal successfully, without any screw failures or screw removals. Caterini and colleagues[26] performed fusion procedures on 51 toes using the cannulated screw, and found bony union in 48 toes. The remaining toes had asymptomatic nonunions. However, 7 screws required removal because of persistent pain from the screw head at the distal digital tuft.

Ellington and colleagues[28] performed arthrodesis on 38 toes using the 2-component intramedullary screw, and reported fusion in 61%; however, successful alignment was maintained in 82%. Witt and Hyer[29] reported on a newer single-component intramedullary device in 7 toes and found good alignment, 100% bony union, and no cases of implant failure or implant migration. Each patient related a decrease in preoperative pain and cosmesis, and was willing to recommend the procedure to a friend. Angirasa and colleagues[30] performed a retrospective analysis of 28 patients and compared a

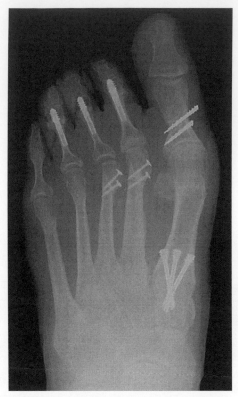

Fig. 5. Radiograph taken 5 years postoperatively. Note the presence of the intramedullary digital fusion devices, which have achieved excellent fusion.

titanium-nickel implant with Kirschner-wire fixation of digital arthrodesis. The intramedullary nickel-titanium device was found to be superior to Kirschner wire in terms of pain, complications, and return to work status. The investigators also noted a significant number of complications in the Kirschner-wire group and none in the intramedullary device group. Delmi[36] reported use of the SmartToe in 170 toes, and achieved fusion in 167 toes at 12-month follow-up.

SUMMARY

Deformities of the lesser digits, including hammer toes, mallet toes, and claw toes, are among the most frequent complaints treated by the foot and ankle surgeon. Arthrodesis of the digit offers good long-term correction and predictability. End-to-end fusion of the PIP joint with Kirschner-wire fixation is most commonly performed; however, this offers stability in only one plane and leaves exposed hardware, with its associated complications. Newer implants currently in use are innovative, and take advantage of the latest metallurgic and polymeric advances. Although newer implants are more expensive and are slightly more difficult to insert than Kirschner wires, they provide good stability, no percutaneous wires, comparable rates of fusion, decreased rates of infection, and increased patient satisfaction. Therefore, the foot and ankle surgeon should consider these newer devices when making a choice for hammer-toe correction.

REFERENCES

1. Ellington JK. Hammertoes and clawtoes: proximal interphalangeal joint correction. Foot Ankle Clin 2011;16:547–58.
2. Soule RE. Operation for the correction of hammer toe. N Y Med J 1910;84: 649–50.
3. Higgs SL. Hammer-toe. Presse Med 1931;131:473–4.
4. Young CS. An operation for the correction of hammer toe and claw-toe. J Bone Joint Surg 1938;20(3):715–9.
5. Taylor RG. An operative procedure for the treatment of hammer toe and claw toe. J Bone Joint Surg 1940;22(3):608–9.
6. Schuberth JM. Preferred practice guidelines: hammer toe syndrome. J Foot Ankle Surg 1999;38(2):166–78.
7. Good J, Fiala K. Digital surgery: current trends and techniques. Clin Podiatr Med Surg 2010;27:583–99.
8. Chadwick C, Saxby TS. Hammertoes/clawtoes: metatarsophalangeal joint correction. Foot Ankle Clin 2011;16:559–71.
9. Coughlin MJ, Dorris J, Polk E. Operative repair of the fixed hammertoe deformity. Foot Ankle Int 2000;21(2):94–104.
10. D'Angelantonio AM, Nelson-Rinaldi KA, Barnard J, et al. Master techniques in digital arthrodesis. Clin Podiatr Med Surg 2012;29:21–40.
11. Lehman DE, Smith RW. Treatment of symptomatic hammertoe with a proximal interphalangeal joint arthrodesis. Foot Ankle Int 1995;16:535–41.
12. Miller JM, Blacklidge DK, Ferdowsian V, et al. Chevron arthrodesis of the interphalangeal joint for hammertoe correction. J Foot Ankle Surg 2010;49:194–6.
13. Weil LS Jr. Hammertoe arthrodesis using conical reamers and internal pin fixation. J Foot Ankle Surg 1999;38(5):370–1.
14. Alvine FG, Garwin KL. Peg and dowel fusion of the proximal interphalangeal joint. Foot Ankle 1980;1:90.
15. Winemaker MJ, Amendola A. Comparison of bioabsorbable pins and Kirschner wires in the fixation of chevron osteotomies for hallux valgus. Foot Ankle Int 1996;17:623–8.
16. Raikin SM, Ching AC. Bioabsorbable fixation in foot and ankle. Foot Ankle Clin 2005;10:667–84.
17. Yu GV, Vincent A, Khoury W. Exploring new advances in digital arthrodesis. Podiatry Today 2003;16(9):40–54.
18. Ford TC, Maurer LM, Myrick KW. Cortical bone pin fixation: a preliminary report on fixation of digital arthrodeses and distal chevron first metatarsal osteotomies. J Foot Ankle Surg 2002;41(1):23–9.
19. Burchardt H. The biology of bone graft repair. Clin Orthop Relat Res 1983;174: 28–42.
20. Vanore JV. Implants. In: Banks AS, Downey MS, Martin DE, et al, editors. McGlamry's forefoot surgery. 1st edition. Philadelphia: Lippincott Williams and Wilkins; 2004. p. 173–4.
21. Fernandez DJ, Perez RV, Medes AM, et al. Understanding the shape-memory alloys used in orthodontics. ISRN Dent 2011;2011:132408.
22. Harris W IV, Mote GA, Malay DS. Fixation of the proximal interphalangeal arthrodesis with the use of an intraosseous loop of stainless-steel wire suture. J Foot Ankle Surg 2009;48(3):411–4.
23. Vanik RK, Weber RC, Matloub HS, et al. The comparative strengths of internal fixation techniques. J Hand Surg Am 1984;9(2):216–21.

24. Halpern FP, Trepal MJ, Hodge W. Contamination and infection rate of percutaneous Kirschner wires in foot surgery. J Am Podiatr Med Assoc 1990;80(8): 433–7.

25. Reese AT, Stone NH, Young AB. Toe fusion using Kirschner wire: a study of the postoperative infection rate and related problems. J R Coll Surg Edinb 1987; 32(3):158–63.

26. Caterini R, Farsetti P, Tarantino U, et al. Arthrodesis of the toe joints with an intramedullary cannulated screw for correction of hammertoe deformity. Foot Ankle Int 2004;25(4):256–61.

27. Lane GD. Lesser digital fusion with a cannulated screw. J Foot Ankle Surg 2005; 44(2):172–3.

28. Ellington JK, Anderson RB, Davis WH, et al. Radiographic analysis of proximal interphalangeal joint arthrodesis with an intramedullary fusion device for lesser toe deformities. Foot Ankle Int 2010;31(5):372–6.

29. Witt BL, Hyer CF. Treatment of hammertoe deformity using a one-piece intramedullary device: a case series. J Foot Ankle Surg 2012;51:450–6.

30. Angirasa AK, Barrett MJ, Silvester D. SmartToe implant compared with Kirschner wire fixation for hammer digit corrective surgery: a review of 28 patients. J Foot Ankle Surg 2012;51(6):711–3.

31. Konkel KF, Sover ER, Menger AG, et al. Hammertoe correction using an absorbable pin. Foot Ankle Int 2011;32(10):973–8.

32. Edwards WH, Beischer AD. Interphalangeal joint arthrodesis of the lesser toes. Foot Ankle Clin 2002;7:43–8.

33. Coughlin MJ. Lesser toe deformities. In: Coughlin MJ, Mann RA, Saltzman CL, editors. Surgery of the foot and ankle, vol. 1, 8th edition. Philadelphia: Mosby Elsevier; 2007. p. 363–464.

34. Miller SJ. Hammer toe correction by arthrodesis of the proximal interphalangeal joint using cortical bone allograft pin. J Am Podiatr Med Assoc 2002;92:563–9.

35. Konkel KF, Menger AG, Retzlaff SA. Hammer toe correction using an absorbable intramedullary pin. Foot Ankle Int 2007;28(8):916–20.

36. Delmi M. Hammer toe surgical correction. Available at: http://www.mmi-usa.com/pdf/hammertoe.pdf. Accessed November 4, 12.

Absorbable Fixation in Forefoot Surgery
A Viable Alternative to Metallic Hardware

David L. Nielson, DPM[a,*], Nathan J. Young, DPM, AACFAS, AAFAS[a,b],
Charles M. Zelen, DPM, FACFAS, FACFAOM[a,b]

KEYWORDS

- Absorbable fixation • ORIF • Polylactic acid • Polyglycolic acid • Polydiaxonone
- Tornier RFS screw

KEY POINTS

- Absorbable fixation has progressed to become a reliable, cost-effective alternative to metallic hardware.
- Newer absorbable devices have been formulated to provide adequate strength for healing and a smooth degradation to limit the local inflammation typically associated with first-generation devices.
- Historically, fixation with absorbable devices can be time-consuming due to a more difficult insertion; however, new innovative technologies to aid in the insertion of these devices are now becoming more common in the orthopedic realm.

INTRODUCTION

Bone repair has been divided into the following 4 stages: inflammation, soft callus formation, hard callus formation, and remodeling. The inflammatory stage begins immediately following the trauma to within hours after trauma. Disruption of the blood supply leads to hematoma formation recruitment of inflammatory cells to slowly resorb the hematoma and the devitalized bone. This localized inflammation exhibits the classic signs of inflammation, including calor, dolor, tumor, palor, and functio laesa. Next, soft callus is formed after an infiltration of fibrous tissue and chondroblasts surrounding the fracture site, which replace the hematoma. This structural network promotes stability across the injured bone as a type of temporary fixation. The callus becomes harder and denser and the fracture site is filled with bone matrix. Once

[a] Foot and Ankle Associates of Southwest Virginia, 1802 Braeburn Drive, Suite M120, Salem, VA 24153, USA; [b] Professional Education and Research Institute, 222 Walnut Avenue, Roanoke, VA 24016, USA
* Corresponding author.
E-mail address: david.l.nielson@gmail.com

Clin Podiatr Med Surg 30 (2013) 283–293
http://dx.doi.org/10.1016/j.cpm.2013.04.001
0891-8422/13/$ – see front matter © 2013 Published by Elsevier Inc.

podiatric.theclinics.com

the bone has united the fracture site, the remodeling phase begins. Fibrous bone is eventually replaced by lamellar bone. This process is known as secondary healing and exists when there is a large gap in the fracture site or there is movement in the fracture site.

Primary bone healing is accomplished when the fracture/osteotomy is held tightly together with anatomic approximation. When this is the case, the formation of callus is essentially skipped because there is no need for stabilization. Mesenchymal cells from the bone marrow are recruited and function as osteoclasts, which will form cutting cones across the fracture site. Capillary budding then occurs within the cone and allows osteoblasts to line the cone walls and lay down newly formed bone.

The bony union that forms at the end of reparative phase can result in strength equal to or greater than that of intact bone before surgery or before injury. Therefore, internal fixation is useful until trabeculation has crossed the fracture site and bony union is formed, typically taking from 4 to 8 weeks. Therefore, the presence of internal fixation is most important through the healing phase, after which time, there is no longer a need for internal fixation. This leads to one of the strongest reasons to use absorbable fixation.

Absorbable materials for surgery have been used since at least the second century as evidenced by Galen's description of the use of gut suture. However, only in recent decades have modern absorbable materials gained in popularity. Modern bioabsorbable implantation began in the early 1960s with the development of the absorbable sutures Dexon (polyglycolic acid, or PGA) and later Vicryl (a copolymer of PGA and polylactic acid, or PLA) and PDS (polydioxanone).[1] Bioabsorbable screws were subsequently developed and were first implanted for use in internal fixation and ligament repair in 1984,[2] but were not commercially available in the United States until 1991. Since that time, the implants have been used with increasing frequency for the fixation of fractures and osteotomies.

Metallic hardware has been the mainstay for the fixation of fractures, osteotomies, and arthrodeses in the past because of their high strength, low reactivity rates, and relatively low expense. Metallic implants, however, do have their share of shortcomings. Metallic implants are considerably stiffer than bone, which can cause osteopenia due to stress shielding. A second surgery may be required for removal of the hardware, which exposes the patient to further surgical risks and expense.[3] Another disadvantage is that metallic implants are radiopaque, which can make computed tomography and magnetic resonance imaging (MRI) studies less efficacious and impair the imaging of that body part.

Absorbable implants seek to overcome these disadvantages. Bioabsorbable implants theoretically prevent stress shielding because the implants will slowly be hydrolyzed and weakened gradually, thus transferring the load to the healing bone, which can lead to normal bone remodeling and normal bone density.[4,5] Bioabsorbable implants eliminate the need of a second surgery for hardware removal. Bioabsorbable implants are radiolucent, which will improve the ability to assess bone healing radiographically. In addition, Rokkanen and colleagues[6] reviewed more than 2500 surgical cases involving bioabsorbable implants and found a decreased risk of infection, which may be due to the hydrolysis of the implants because they degrade, which creates an environment whereby bacteria cannot proliferate and therefore make infection unlikely to occur.

Naturally, there are shortcomings to bioabsorbable implants as well. The strength of bioabsorbable implants is inferior to metallic implants and as such is not indicated for fixation of fractures, which require a high degree of interfragmentary compression. Although they are weaker than stainless steel implants, numerous biomechanical studies have shown that bioabsorble implants' strength exceeds the physiologic loads for many applications and are therefore sufficient and appropriate in such situations.[5,7] Bioabsorbable implants that are placed under greater loads tend to degrade faster and are therefore not indicated in the bridging of bony deficits or in severely comminuted fractures.[5,8]

Bioabsorbable implants are typically more expensive than metallic implants. However, there is a cost savings when used in applications whereby hardware removal is frequently performed because the need for a second surgery would be eliminated.[4] Inflammatory reactions and osteolysis have been reported in the literature for bioabsorbable implants.[9] The reactions are clinically manifested as local pain, redness, swelling, fluid accumulation or sterile sinus formation, osteolysis, or pronounced fibrous encapsulation.[5,7,9] These adverse reactions are thought to be due to the rapid rate of degradation of the implant with local accumulation of breakdown products outpacing the local tissue's ability to clear them. However, according to Winemaker and Amendola,[10] this seems to be more of a problem with larger implants being used in larger bones and with earlier generation implants. Newer implants have a lower risk of such adverse reactions because of their smoother resorption characteristics.

Bioabsorbable implants are best used in situations associated with low load, the anticipation of rapid healing, and for the fixation of small bone fragments.[11] In the foot and ankle, proven indications for the use of bioabsorbable implants include the fixation of syndesmotic injuries, Lisfranc injuries, osteochondral defects, tendon transfers,[7] and first metatarsal chevron osteotomy.[2,9–15] They should be used with great caution and are relatively contraindicated in morbidly obese patients, patients with compromised healing potential secondary to advanced age, immunosupression, diabetes, or smoking, or in the noncompliant patient.[4,9,13] Obesity increases the load on the implant, which tends to cause more rapid degradation of the implant, possibly due to microfractures, and will likely cause failure of the implant.[8]

The benefits of bioabsorbable implants have only recently come to the forefront in orthopedics because of improvements in polymer science. Bioabsorbable implants are chains of covalently bonded subunits (monomers) that form a polymer.[8] The subunits forming the chemical structure of the biabsorbable polymer are composed of lactic acid, glycolic acid, or para-dioxanone. These monomers are then covalently joined to either similar or dissimilar monomers, forming long polymer chains. A chain that is composed of a single repeating subunit is a homopolymer, whereas a chain composed of a combination of subunits is a copolymer. PGA and PLA are examples of homopolymers.[3] The combination PGA and PLA copolymer seeks to take advantage of the strength of PGA and the lower reactivity of PLA.

These bioabsorbable polymeric chains are degraded locally through enzymatic hydrolysis into their monomeric subunits, which may then be further hydrolyzed via the Krebs cycle into water and carbon dioxide. The final breakdown products are then excreted through the lungs with some intermediate breakdown products being excreted through the kidneys.[1,3] The rate of hydrolysis is affected by the implant's chemical composition, its crystalline or amorphous structure, the manufacturing process, the sterilization process, its physical dimensions, and the site at which it is implanted.[5] The rate of hydrolysis may cause localized inflammation if the breakdown overwhelms the local tissue's ability to dispose of these products, which can lead to edema and, in some instances, a sterile sinus, osteolysis, or even encapsulation.[6,9]

The bioabsorbable implants that are commercially available are polylactic acid and its isomers, polyglycolic acid, polydiaxone, or copolymers of the above. Each monomer has distinct characteristics that dictate the molecule's rigidity and degradation. Crystalline structures tend to have increased tensile strength and longer degradation processes when compared with amorphous structures.[7] Hydrophilic structures tend to be hydrolyzed more rapidly than hydrophobic structures. Some structures are asymmetrical and have different isomers, which will have different properties.

Lactic acid is a hydrophobic, asymmetrical 3-carbon molecule. Because it is hydrophobic, it tends to degrade much slower than the hydrophilic materials. Because it is asymmetrical, it can be found in both a levo and a dextro isomer. The polymerized isomers of lactic acid will form poly-L-lactic acid (PLLA) or poly-DL-lactic acid. The levo isomer forms a crystalline structure, whereas the dextro isomer forms an amorphous structure. This difference in structure greatly influences the respective isomers' strength and degradation profile. For example, the strength profile of self-reinforced PLLA pins decreases to the level of cancellous bone in 36 weeks and is present in bone for up to 5 years.[5] However, when the amorphous enantiomer is added, the combination of the 2 stereoisomers forms a copolymer with a strength and degradation profile somewhere between the 2 monomers, depending on its composition.[8]

Polyglycolic acid is a hard, crystalline molecule that is hydrophilic in nature. In fact, PGA has the highest initial mechanical properties. Due to PGA's hydrophilic nature, it is quickly hydrolyzed and is degraded very rapidly, causing PGA implants to lose one-half of its initial bending and shear strength within 1 to 2 weeks and may even cause a clinical foreign body reaction, which is usually evident between 8 and 16 weeks.[16] Due to its rapid hydrolyzation, PGA is rarely used by itself currently; it is frequently used in combination with other absorbable implants, specifically PLLA.

Polydiaxone is produced by polymerizing the monomer para-diaxone. The polymer's structure is inherently stiff and is commonly used in sutures and pins. PDS loses strength in 4 to 6 weeks.[9,12] Multiple studies have successfully used PDS pins in the correction of hallux valgus.[12,14,15]

In an effort to find a balance between a material's strength profile and degradation rate, combinations of the materials have been developed. The biomechanical and biochemical properties of a copolymer differs from those of its constituent monomers[8] and by altering the composition of each monomer, the rate of degradation, and the biomechanical properties can be manipulated.[7,17] For example, the PLLA and PGA copolymer seeks the greater strength of PGA and the slower degradation and reactivity rates of PLLA. This combination of polymers maintains its mechanical strength for at least 8 weeks and is fully resorbed within approximately 24 months.[5]

There are many bioabsorbable devices that have been developed for surgical use. These devices include sutures, pins, staples, screws, suture anchors, interference screws, and plates. Some of these devices are no longer in use or have limited use in the foot and ankle. For example, sutures are rarely, if ever, used to fixate osteotomies in the foot and ankle, despite the fact that Lapidus and Mitchell both originally described their eponymous osteomies being fixated with absorbable suture. Bioabsorbable staples are not available in the United States for fixation of bone. For completeness, however, these devices will be reviewed briefly.

Bioabsorbable suture was the first artificial bioabsorbable surgical device developed. Artificial bioabsorbable surgical sutures have been in wide use since the 1960s. Dexon (PGA), Vicryl (PLLA and PGA copolymer), and PDS sutures are all frequently used for soft tissue closure and rarely for bony fixation. With advancements in Albeight gen shaften (AO) principles, rigid internal and/or external fixation is more commonly used. Biomechanical studies have shown that the stainless steel screws are 4 times stronger and are 12 times more stable than suture fixation. In a prospective, randomized trial, Calder and colleagues compared the use of suture fixation to screw fixation in the Mitchell procedure. They found that patients who underwent fixation by suture returned to their regular shoe gear, social activities, and employment significantly later than those who underwent fixation by screws. The suture group also had a lower degree of patient satisfaction. Calder and colleagues[18] reported that the prolonged immobilization period following suture fixation is unacceptable in such a common procedure. One recent development in the use of bioabsorbable suture for skin closure is closure using barbed suture. Gililland and colleagues[19] found that the use of barbed sutures in the closure of total knee arthroplasties compared with a standard interrupted suture technique was 2.3 minutes faster; the closure cost was similar, and the perioperative complication rates were similar. The use of barbed suture in foot and ankle surgery may be limited.

Tapered and straight pins are available in many different polymer/copolymer forms. In the foot and ankle, tapered pins are primarily used to repair osteochondral defects of the talus, and historically in chevron ostetomies, although straight pins are primarily used in digital arthroplasty/arthrodesis. Other applications might include pediatric fracture fixation, intra-articular fracture fixation, and crossing pins for stable fractures or osteotomies. Straight pins offer very little compression. Tapered pins offer increased compression when compared with straight pins, but meager compression when compared with other forms of fixation. They are therefore not indicated in the fixation of a fracture or osteotomy where significant compression and stability is required.

Although not available in the United States, absorbable staples have been developed and are used internationally. PLLA staples were originally developed for the treatment of carpal-scaphoid fractures.[20] In a study conducted by Barca and Busa, PLLA staples were used to fixate 25 Akin osteotomies. They found 24 of 25 of the osteotomies (96%) were healed within 5 weeks and the remaining osteotomy in a patient with juvenile diabetes was healed at 12 weeks with no deformity. A single staple was used in 28% of the cases; however, 2 staples were required in 72% of the cases.[21] Osteo-tec (Montpellier, France) has developed a Poly-D-lactide and Poly-L-lactide (P-D/L-LA) steroisomer copolymer compression staple, the Aros MF, for the use of metatarsal and phalangeal osteotomies. This device is unfortunately not available in the United States. To the best of the authors' knowledge, there are currently no absorbable staples for bony fixation available in the United States at this time.

There are absorbable staples for the use of subcuticular skin closure currently available in the United States. Insorb staples (Incisive Surgical, Plymouth, MN, USA) are horizontal subcuticular staples composed of a copolymer of PLA and PGA. This device may help to speed wound closure after surgery and to offer better cosmesis due to the lack of percutaneous entry of the closure method. In a prospective study conducted by Cross and colleagues[22] and reported in the journal of *Plastic and Reconstructive Surgery* in 2009, it was found that the PLA/PGA copolymer subcuticular staple device allowed their surgical wounds to be closed 4 times faster than standard suture closing techniques with decreased inflammation and equivocal scarring. These staples have found wider use in general, plastic, and obstetric/gynecologic surgery, but are also indicated in orthopedic surgery. The foot and ankle offer few opportunities to use the device because it is contraindicated in tissue that is too thin or too thick to allow adequate capture of the device; however, one potential indication in foot and ankle surgery for which this technology may be of benefit is in the soft tissue closure following gastrocnemius recession.

Bioabsorbable screws are produced by many companies and come in a variety compositions and sizes. Bioabsorbable screws offer increased compression across an osteotomy or fracture, but are still much less compressive than their stainless steel and titanium counterparts. As such, bioabsorbable screws are indicated in areas that are stable with very low loads. Indications for absorbable screws in the foot and ankle include syndesmotic ruptures, Lis Franc injuries, and Akin and Austin osteotomies. The screws are often time consuming to insert when compared with modern stainless steel and titanium screws that are cannulated, self-drilling, and self-tapping.

One area of emerging research regarding bioabsorbable implants involves the use of ultrasonic energy that semi-liquefies the polymer. This welds the implant into bone and forms a rivet on the distal end of the implant.[23] Biomechanical tests have found that a device implanted with ultrasonic energy has up to 11.5 times the tensile strength and stiffness of a similarly composed nonultrasonic screw.[24] The major advantage of this method is the ease and speed of application when compared with nonultrasonic screws. The technology has been in use in craniomaxillofacial surgery for some time with some early research available.[25] Newer applications of this technology in noncraniomaxillofacial surgery are only beginning to be realized.

Bioabsorbable plates have been long used in craniomaxillofacial surgery and also in hand surgery in Europe.[7] Bioabsorbable plates have good conforming properties, which are important in craniomaxillofacial surgery. These types of absorbable plates are available for foot and ankle use; however, the plates provide inadequate strength and stability to be useful on a regular basis in the lower extremities.

Bioabsorbable interference screws and suture anchors are available from many orthopedic companies in many sizes and materials. Many tendon transfers of the foot and ankle involve the transfer a tendon through a bone tunnel. Bioabsorbable interference screws are beneficial for this application if there is concern about

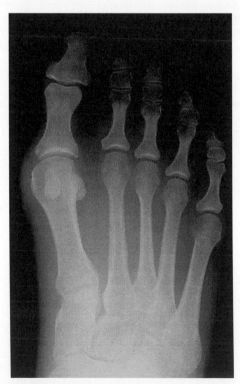

Fig. 1. Preoperative radiograph revealing moderate increase in the first intermetatarsal angle, moderately increased distal articular set angle, and a hypertrophic first metatarsal head with enlarged medial prominence.

postoperative MRI visualization. In a study regarding anterior cruciate ligament repair, it was found that bioabsorbable interference screw performance was equivocal to that of metal screws.[26] Suture anchors are widely used in foot and ankle surgery for the reattachment of the Achilles tendon after saucerization of calcaneal bone or debridement of tendon and for the reconstruction of the lateral ankle ligaments in Broström and Broström-Gould procedures. Absorbable implants are an effective alternative to metal implants if there is concern about migration into a joint or postoperative MRI visualization difficulty.

Although there are many varieties of resorbable implants for many indications in the lower extremities, resorbable fixation is most widely accepted for the fixation of the first ray. The following is a case example of the copolymer PLGA 85/15 (RFS screw from Tornier, Edina, MN, USA), which offers great initial strength and smooth resorption over 18 to 24 months.

PATIENT HISTORY

This 40-year-old patient presented to the clinic for evaluation of her significant hallux valgus deformity. The patient is a health care worker and specifically requested absorbable fixation after her own personal appropriate care of her deformity. The

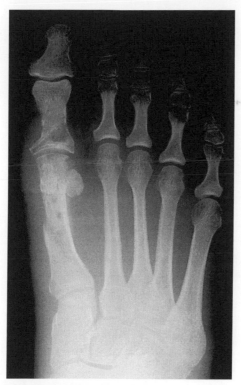

Fig. 2. Three months status post Austin Akin double osteotomy. Note the improved alignment of the hallux. Note also the screw holes from the resorbable fixation device are visible at this time.

patient had the bunion for several years. She failed substantial conservative care and opted for surgery.

PHYSICAL EXAMINATION

The patient had palpable pedal pulses, capillary refill time 2 to 3 seconds, and no pallor on elevation. Sharp and dull and light touch sensations are intact. Protective threshold is intact. Proprioception was intact. The patient exhibited normal color, turgor, and texture of her foot with the exception of the first metatarsophalangeal joint (MTPJ), which was mildly edematous and erythematous. She was noted to have hallux valgus deformity, right greater than left, with dorsomedial bony prominence. She had good range of motion and muscle strength 5/5.

IMAGING AND ADDITIONAL TESTING

Three views of the right foot do show a moderate bunion deformity with a moderate amount of hallux abductovalgus and medial bunion prominence. The first intermetatarsal angle was 13° and the hallux valgus angle was 23° (**Fig. 1**).

CASE DISCUSSION

A case of the correction of hallux valgus using a Tornier RFS screw is presented. The RFS screw is a copolymer of PLLA and PGA in an 85% to 15% mix, respectively. This

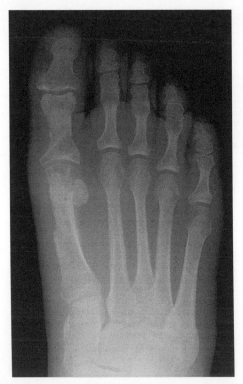

Fig. 3. Six months status post Austin Akin double osteotomy. Note the improved alignment of the hallux. Note also the screw holes from the resorbable fixation device are becoming less visible at this time.

ratio is used to achieve the greatest benefit of PGA's strength with the lower reactivity rates of PLLA. This copolymer maintains its mechanical strength for at least 8 weeks and is fully resorbed within approximately 18 to 24 months.

Attention was directed to the dorsomedial aspect of the patient's foot where a 6-cm longitudinal incision was made parallel to the extensor hallucis longus and involved the contour of the deformity. Dissection was performed in layers. The periosteum was dissected using a Colorado tip on the Bovie device, which is excellent at stripping the periosteum from the bone. Next, the hypertrophy on the medial aspect of the first metatarsal head was removed using a sagittal saw. Attention was then directed to the first interspace where a release of the conjoint tendon and lateral capsulotomy was performed. Attention was then redirected medially where a long arm chevron osteotomy was made in the center of the first metatarsal head. Once osteotomized, the head was shifted laterally and impacted on the proximal part of the metatarsal in its corrected position. Once in its corrected position, the osteotomy was stabilized using guide wires. A thread hole was drilled followed by a proximal over drill for compression, and then a tap. Once prepared, an RFS screw was inserted into each of the screw holes. The excess absorbable screw on the near and far cortices was removed and contoured using a high-temperature cautery device. The medial bone shelf was then removed. It was noted at this time that the patient still had a moderate amount of hallux valgus because of her distal articular set angle and it was decided to continue with an Akin osteotomy. Once the periosteum was freed from the proximal phalanx, an

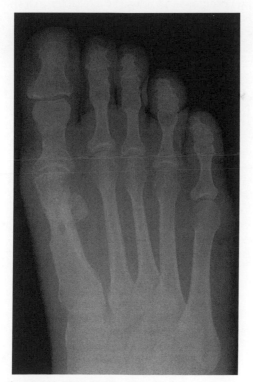

Fig. 4. Eighteen months status post Austin Akin double osteotomy. Note the improved alignment of the hallux and the well-preserved first MTPJ space. Note also the screw holes from the resorbable fixation device are less visible at this time.

oblique closing wedge osteotomy was performed on the proximal phalanx with the lateral cortical hinge left intact. Once in its corrected position, the osteotomy was stabilized using guide wires. A thread hole was drilled followed by a proximal over drill for compression, and then a tap. Once prepared, an RFS screw was inserted into each of the screw holes. At this time it was noted that the patient's preoperative deformity was corrected and the capsule and skin were closed in layers. The foot was dressed in dry sterile dressing and a well-padded postoperative splint was applied.

Postoperatively the patient exhibited minimal edema and erythema. This edema and erythema were similar to the edema and erythema present after a bunion procedure fixated using nonbioabsorbable hardware. The patient was kept in a splint and then cast for approximately 2 and one-half weeks and then transitioned to a cam boot. At 6 weeks' postoperatively, radiographs revealed excellent alignment, solid bony union, and no peri-implant osteolysis. Subjectively the patient was extremely pleased with the alignment and the outcome of the procedure. She was followed for 18 months. Her 3-month, 6-month, and 18-month radiographs all show excellent alignment, solid bony fusion, well-preserved first MTPJ joint space, and no osteolysis (**Figs. 2–4**). At the 18-month radiograph, most of the bioabsorbable implants were no longer visible. The first intermetatarsal angle was measured at 8° and the hallux valgus angle was measured at 13° at 18 months postoperatively (see **Fig. 4**).

SUMMARY

Absorbable fixation has progressed to become a reliable, cost-effective alternative to metallic hardware. Older generation absorbable devices hydrolyzed faster than the tissue was able to process and used reactive dyes and, as a result, the earlier devices were associated with large inflammatory reactions with drainage. Newer devices have been formulated to prevent these complications. Newer resorbable devices have very low rates of reactivity.

REFERENCES

1. Wood GW II. General principles of fracture treatment. In: Canale ST, Beaty JH, editors. Canale and Beaty: Campbell's operative orthopedics. 11th edition. Philadelphia: Mosby Elsevier; 2008. p. 3048–9.
2. Pelto-Vasenius K, Hirvensalo E, Vasenius J, et al. Osteolytic changes afer polyglycolide pin fixation in chevron osteotomy. Foot Ankle Int 1997;18:21–5.
3. Hollinger JO, Battistone GC. Biodegradable bone repair materials. Synthetic polymers and ceramics. Clin Orthop Relat Res 1986;(207):290–305.
4. Hovis WD, Kaiser BW, Watson JT, et al. Treatment of syndesmotic disruptions of the ankle with bioabsorbable screw fixation. J Bone Joint Surg Am 2002;84: 26–31.
5. Waris E, Konttinen Y, Ashammakhi N, et al. Bioabsorbable fixation devies in trauma and bone surgery: current clinical standing. Expert Rev Med Devices 2004;1(2):229–40.
6. Rokkanen P, Böstman O, Vainionpää S, et al. Absorbable devices in the fixation of fractures. J Trauma 1996;40:S123–7.
7. Raikin SM, Ching AC. Bioabsorbable fixation in foot and ankle. Foot Ankle Clin 2005;10:667–84.
8. Ciccone WJ 2nd, Motz C, Bentley C, et al. Bioabsorbable implants in orthopaedics: new developments and clinical applications. J Am Acad Orthop Surg 2001;5:280–8.

9. Caminear DS, Pavlovich R Jr, Peitrzak WS. Fixation of the chevron osteotomy with an absorbable copolymer pin for treatment of hallux valgus deformity. J Foot Ankle Surg 2005;44:203–10.

10. Winemaker MJ, Amendola A. Comparison of bioabsorbable pins and Kirschner wires in the fixation of chevron osteomtomies for hallux valgus. Foot Ankle Int 1996;17:623–8.

11. Gill LH, Martin DF, Coumas JM, et al. Fixation with bioabsorbable pins in chevron bunionectomy. J Bone Joint Surg Am 1997;79:1510–8.

12. Alcelik I, Alnaib M, Pollock R, et al. Bioabsorbable fixation for Mitchell's bunion-ectomy osteotomy. J Foot Ankle Surg 2009;48:9–14.

13. Barca F, Busa R. Austin/Chevron osteotomy fixed with bioabsorbable poly-L-lactic acid single screw. J Foot Ankle Surg 1997;36:15–20.

14. DeOrio JK, Ware AW. Single absorbable polydioxanone pin fixation for distal chevron bunion osteotomies. Foot Ankle Int 2001;22:832–5.

15. Small HN, Braly WG, Tullos HS. Fixation of the Chevron osteotomy utilizing absorbable polydioxanon pins. Foot Ankle Int 1995;16:346–50.

16. Rokkanen P, Böstman O, Hirvensalo E, et al. Bioabsorbable fixation in orthopaedic surgery and traumatology. Biomaterials 2000;21:2607–13.

17. Spitalney DA. Bioabsorbable implants. Clin Podiatr Med Surg 2006;23:673–94.

18. Calder JD, Holligdale JP, Pearse MF. Screw versus suture fixation of Mitchell's osteotomy: a prospective, randomised study. J Bone Joint Surg Br 1999;81(4):621–4.

19. Gililland JM, Anderson LA, Sun G, et al. Perioperative closure-related complication rates and cost analysis of barbed suture for closure in TKA. Clin Orthop Relat Res 2012;470(1):125–9.

20. Bedeschi P. Osteosynthesis of the carpal scaphoid with mini-bioabsorbable staples. In: Vastamaki M, editor. Current trends in hand surgery. Amsterdam: Elsevier; 1995. p. 79–83.

21. Barca F, Busa R. Resorbable poly-L-lactic acid mini-staples for the fixation of Akin osteotomies. J Foot Ankle Surg 1997;36:106–11.

22. Cross KJ, Teo EH, Wong SJ, et al. The absorbable dermal staple device: a faster, more cost-effective method for incisional closure. Plast Reconstr Surg 2009;124(1):156–62.

23. Abdulazim A, Penzkofer R, Wipf F, et al. Paper 28: ultrasonic welding of bio-absorbablepins in cancellous bone for fracture fixation. J Bone Joint Surg Br 2010;92-B(Suppl I):75.

24. Buijs GJ, van der Houwen EB, Stegenga B, et al. Mechanical strength and stiffness of the biodegradable SonicWeld Rx osteofixation system. J Oral Maxillofac Surg 2009;67(4):782–7.

25. Meara DJ, Knoll MR, Holmes JD, et al. Fixation of Le Fort I osteotomies with poly-DL-lactic acid mesh and ultrasonic welding – a new technique. J Oral Maxillofac Surg 2012;70(5):1139–44.

26. Płomiński J, Borcz K, Kwiatkowski K, et al. Fixation of patellar tendon bone graft in reconstruction of patellar ligaments. Comparison of bioabsorbable and metal interference screws—results of treatment. Ortop Traumatol Rehabil 2008;10(1):44–53.

Alternative Methods in Fixation for Capital Osteotomies in Hallux Valgus Surgery

Charles M. Zelen, DPM, FACFAS, FACFAOM*,
Nathan J. Young, DPM, AACFAS, AAFAS

KEYWORDS

- Hallux abducto valgus • Austin bunionectomy • Chevron osteotomy
- Stryker Sonic Fusion bioresorbable pin

KEY POINTS

- Capital osteotomies of the first metatarsal remain a tested method for the correction of hallux valgus.
- As the osteotomies have evolved, so too have the fixation options.
- Current research and development of implant devices is leading to implants that (1) provide increased strength and stability; (2) are easier to implant, thus reducing operative time; and/or (3) bioabsorbable implants with a chemical profile that provides smoother absorption to give adequate strength and lower reactivity.

INTRODUCTION

Hallux valgus is one of the most frequent disorders encountered by the foot and ankle specialist. Although the exact prevalence of hallux valgus is unknown, it is estimated to be in the realm of 23% for persons aged 18 to 65 years with prevalence increasing in the elderly and in women.[1] Many factors may influence the progression of the deformity, such as abnormal biomechanics, abnormal anatomy, joint hypermobility, or the presence of an inflammatory joint condition. Diagnosis is frequently obvious in the clinical setting, with an enlarged dorsomedial bony prominence at the first metatarsal phalangeal joint (MTPJ). However, hallux valgus is typically diagnosed by measuring the first intermetatarsal angle and the hallux valgus angle using weight-bearing radiographs. The values of these measurements should be 8° to 12° for a normal intermetatarsal angle and approximately 15° or less for the hallux valgus angle.

Treatment of hallux valgus is varied and is often dependent on the practitioner. In general, long-term conservative treatment of this condition is of little benefit, because

Professional Education and Reseach Institute, 222 Walnut Avenue, Roanoke VA 24016, USA
* Corresponding author. Professional Education and Reseach Institute, 222 Walnut Avenue, Roanoke VA 24016, USA.
E-mail address: cmzelen@periedu.com

Clin Podiatr Med Surg 30 (2013) 295–306
http://dx.doi.org/10.1016/j.cpm.2013.04.002
0891-8422/13/$ – see front matter © 2013 Published by Elsevier Inc.

the deformity often progresses despite reasonable conservative treatment. The American College of Foot and Ankle Surgeons recommends initial conservative treatment before any surgical intervention. Conservative therapies may include shoe modifications, orthoses, splinting, padding, or nonsteroidal antiinflammatory drugs.

There are a multitude of surgeries for the correction of a bunion deformity. Helal[2] counted more than 150 different surgical options more than 30 years ago and the number continues to increase. For small to moderate increases in the first intermetatarsal angle, a distal osteotomy of the metatarsal is usually indicated. The first report of an osteotomy of the first metatarsal for correction of a bunion deformity was in 1881 by Reverdin.[3] He described his osteotomy as a closing wedge osteotomy with the apex laterally so as also to excise the medial bony protuberance. This procedure addresses the proximal articular set angle, but does not address the intermetatarsal angle.

In 1920 Roux[4] described a capital osteotomy for the correction of hallux valgus. This osteotomy removes a trapezoid-shaped wedge from the metatarsal head and leaves a shelf laterally. The first cut of this osteotomy is distal in a dorsal-to-plantar, through-and-through manner in the medial portion of the metatarsal head. The second cut is proximal and transects the metatarsal head. The third cut is made perpendicularly to the first cut and removes the trapezoidal fragment. With the fragment now removed, the head is shifted laterally. The removal of the trapezoidal bone fragment allows correction of the proximal articular set angle, the hallux abductus angle, and the intermetatarsal angle.[5] This osteotomy is similar to the Mitchell osteotomy and its modifications.

Hohmann[6] described an osteotomy in 1921 that is similar to the Reverdin in that a wedge of bone is removed from the metatarsal head. However, the Hohmann procedure has the apex of the wedge not at the far cortex, but rather in the intermetatarsal space. Thus, a trapezoid-shaped bone wedge is resected. Because the osteotomies are through and through, the capital fragment is mobilized and is allowed to move laterally to also decrease the intermetatarsal angle.

Hawkins and colleagues[7] and Mitchell and colleagues[8] described their osteotomy for the correction of hallux valgus in 1945 and again in 1958. This osteotomy is performed by making a distal cut perpendicular to the articular surface in the metatarsal head from dorsal to plantar. The osteotomy does not transect the metatarsal head, instead only one-half to two-thirds of the width of the medial aspect of the metatarsal is transected, depending on the amount of correction required in the intermetatarsal angle. The second osteotomy does transect the metatarsal and is parallel to the distal cut. Next, an osteotomy is made on the capital fragment perpendicular to the first osteotomy to remove a rectangular fragment of bone. The capital fragment is then displaced laterally. The distal cut can be angulated to allow for correction of an increased proximal articular set angle, similar to Roux's[4] description.

The Mitchell osteotomy was originally described using a suture for fixation. In addition, they recommended the use of tongue depressors for splintage for the first 10 days after surgery, followed by a below-knee walking cast for 6 to 8 weeks. Following removal of the below-knee cast, night splints were used for an additional 12 weeks to avoid pressure from the patient's bedclothes.

Wilson[9] described a through-and-through osteotomy of the metatarsal head directed from distal medial to proximal lateral in 1963. However, this osteotomy tends to have increased shortening leading to lesser metatarsalgia; it is inherently less stable than other osteotomies and can lead to malposition of the capital fragment.

Austin and Leventon[10] described their popular V osteotomy of the metatarsal head in 1968 at an American Academy of Orthopedic Surgeons exhibit in Chicago and later published their research in 1981.[11] They described a V osteotomy with the apex at the center of an imaginary circle in the metatarsal head with its bone cuts being horizontally directed at 60°. They reported that this allowed the cuts to be in the cancellous portion of the bone and provided a broad surface of bone contact for better healing.[11]

Johnson and Smith[12] described a derotational, angulational, transpositional osteotomy (DRATO) in 1974. The proximal cut is transverse osteotomy made perpendicular to the shaft at the neck of the metatarsal. The capital fragment is then inverted or everted depending on the rotation present in the hallux. A medial wedge is then resected from the metatarsal by making the second osteotomy parallel to the articular surface, which then realigns the joint. A third osteotomy may be used to plantarflex or dorsiflex the capital fragment. The capital fragment is then transposed laterally to provide correction of the intermetatarsal angle. This technique is rarely used because of its inherent instability and difficulty in fixation.

Many methods of fixation of first metatarsal capital osteotomies have been described in the literature. As the techniques for surgical correction of the deformity have evolved, so too have the stabilization techniques. They include impaction (which technically is not a fixation method), Kirschner wires, sutures, staples, metallic screws, absorbable screws, nonlocking plates, locking plates, and a new hybrid absorbable device.

Austin and Leventon[10] originally described fixation of their V osteotomy by using only hand impaction of the two fragments. They reported that the osteotomy is so stable from the impaction of the soft cancellous fragments that fixation is not necessary. In addition, ground reactive forces should help maintain the impaction during the postoperative period. Hattrup and Johnson[13] performed the Austin bunionectomy on 225 feet and had 4 patients with a displaced metatarsal head (1.8%) and nearly 80% complete satisfaction rate with an additional 12% being satisfied with only minor reservations. In a retrospective study of 100 nonfixated Austin bunionectomy procedures done by Feit and colleagues,[14] they had 1 patient fall and had migration of the capital fragment (1%). All other complication rates were similar to those of fixated Austin bunionectomies. They reported that the nonfixated Austin is an acceptable alternative in hallux valgus surgeries. However, Gudas[15] stated that, in a series of 125 nonfixated procedures, there was a 30% migration rate of the capital fragment, and Jahss and colleagues[16] noted a 12.5% loss of correction. However, Gudas'[15] data were never published. As a result, foot and ankle surgeons have sought many types of internal fixation devices that are easy to use, have low complication rates, and provide sufficient stabilization and/or compression. The original Austin osteotomy has also evolved over time with multiple variations, with the most popular being the Kalish modification that lengthens the dorsal arm so that the osteotomy is more amendable to screw fixation.

Over the last 100 years, hundreds of fixation option have been suggested in the literature, with the first being suture. The Mitchell osteotomy was first described as being held together with suture. Biomechanical studies have shown that the stainless steel screws are 4 times stronger and are 12 times more stable than suture fixation. In a prospective, randomized trial, Calder and colleagues[17] compared the use of suture fixation with screw fixation in the Mitchell procedure. Patients who underwent fixation by suture returned to social activities nearly 3 weeks later than those who underwent fixation by screws. Likewise, the return to work was prolonged by nearly 4 weeks in those in the suture group. The suture group had a lower degree of patient satisfaction at 6 weeks and had a later return to wearing normal footwear. The suture group also had significantly lower forefoot scores at 6 and 12 weeks. The prolonged immobilization period following suture fixation was unacceptable as well.

A newer form of suture fixation uses the use of FiberWire (Arthrex, Naples, FL) to correct the intermetatarsal angle. The FiberWire interosseous suture and a button device are used in the TightRope (Arthrex, Naples, FL) to recreate anatomic ligaments and tendons. Between the first and second metatarsal heads, there is no anatomic ligament to recreate.[18] Therefore, the TightRope device creates an attachment analogous to a ligament that is not present. The device is then tethered down and the intermetatarsal angle is reduced accordingly. The tension placed on the first and second metatarsals can lead to complications. Potential complications of this device include second metatarsal fracture, metatarsalgia, recurrent hallux valgus, and hallux varus. Although this device is an option, further studies should be considered to evaluate the long-term efficacy.

The first metallic fixation considered for hallux valgus repair was stainless steel wire fixation. Multiple forms of wire fixation have been used with the K-wire, or Kirschner wire, being most prevalent. Satisfactory results can be obtained using Kirschner wire fixation. K-wires have the advantage of ease of insertion and removal and limit motion across an osteotomy. K-wires offer good resistance against movement perpendicular to the wire, but offer limited resistance when the motion is parallel to the wire. The wire can be implanted, or it can be inserted percutaneously and removed at a later date. Percutaneous fixation may provide some discomfort to the patient and places the patient at risk for a pin tract infection.

Staples are another fixation option for capital osteotomies. The original description was that the staple simply provided neutralization of the osteotomy without compression but, over the last 15 years, advances have led to creation of staples that compress the osteotomy as well. These compression staples are another alternative for capital fragment fixation and provide adequate compression and allow limited dissection and periosteal disruption. They also offer decreased operating time compared with screws because there are usually fewer steps for the implantation. As such, they may be a reliable alternative for bunion deformity. However, little prospective research has been conducted to review this type of fixation.

The most popular method of fixation of a capital osteotomy is with metallic screws. Screw fixation provides relative stability to an otherwise unstable osteotomy. When inserted in a lag technique, screws can provide compression and, when 2 screws are placed, rotational stability is achieved as well. In stable osteotomies, such as the chevron, a single screw may be efficacious. Modifications of the chevron osteotomy such as the Kalish, with lengthening of the dorsal arm, allow for more correction of the capital fragment and 2 screws for added stability. Piezoelectric studies investigating the shearing forces acting across the first metatarsal during ambulation have shown that screw fixation provides sufficient stability to provide early weight bearing.[17]

Bioresorbable fixation is another alternative for fixation of capital fragment osteotomies. Their main advantage compared with metallic hardware is that metal hardware can back out, become infected, or otherwise cause pain and discomfort and need to be removed. Bioabsorbable screw fixation obviates the second procedure because the implant is fully resorbed in 1 to 4 years. As they degrade over this period, they gradually transfer load to the healing bone and there is no stress shielding. In addition, if imaging studies are needed, there is less scatter or distortion as is see with standard metallic fixation.

The most common usage of bioabsorbable implants in orthopedics is in the chevron osteotomy.[19] Multiple studies have shown that using bioabsorbable implants for the fixation of the distal first metatarsal osteotomy has similar correction of the intermetatarsal angle[19–23] and bony healing and similar complication rates as using other forms of fixation.[20–27]

There are multiple forms of resorbable implants for fixation of capital osteotomies that are available, with the most popular being pins and cannulated screws.

A new development in the surgical treatment of hallux valgus includes the use of a SonicPin (Stryker, Mahwah, NJ). This pin seeks to take advantage of the benefits of both metal and resorbable screw fixation. One area of emerging research regarding bioabsorbable implants involves the use of ultrasonic energy to semiliquefy the polymer, welding the implant into bone and forming a rivet on the distal end of the implant.[28] The technology has been in use in craniomaxillofacial surgery for some time with some early research.[29] Biomechanical tests have found that a device implanted with ultrasonic energy has up to 11.5 times the tensile strength and stiffness of a similarly composed nonultrasonic screw.[30] Newer applications of this technology in noncraniomaxillofacial surgery are only beginning to be realized. In a study conducted by Heiss and colleagues,[31] rabbit femurs were osteotomized and fixated using SonicPins and compared with their control. They found more advanced healing of the osteotomies after 7, 21, 42, and 84 days in the ultrasound-activated resorbable pin groups. The control group fixated with screws had greater stiffness than the ultrasound-activated resorbable pin group. Another biomechanical study conducted by Schneider and colleagues[32] fused 2 blocks of bone using titanium screws and ultrasound-activated resorbable pins. They found equal strength levels of the ultrasonic pins compared with the titanium miniscrews. The major advantage of this method is the ease and speed of application compared with nonultrasonographically implanted absorbable materials. An area of current research with this technology is in hybrid implants, combining metal nails or screws with an ultrasonic absorbable coating that may provide enhanced strength and stiffness and long-term stability.[31] The Sonic Fusion pin (Stryker, Mahwah NJ) is currently indicated for fixation of the Chevron osteotomy (**Figs. 1** and **2**).

Plate and screw constructs have been reported and, most recently, anatomic plates for capital fragment osteotomies have become available. These constructs offer increased stability in multiple planes because the plate is able to withstand increased torsion, compression, and tension forces. Plate and screw constructs increase the surgical time and may increase the dissection and disruption of the periosteum. They may be advantageous in osteoporotic or cystic bone. They may also be beneficial in closing wedge types and less stable osteotomies.[33]

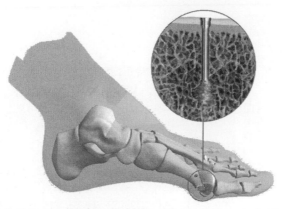

Fig. 1. The Sonic Fusion pin (Stryker, Mahwah, NJ) being inserted. Note on the upper portion of the picture the PLDA material infuses into the surrounding medullary bone after ultrasound charge is applied to fixate the chevron osteotomy. PLDA, Poly Lactic Acid, Dextro anantomer.

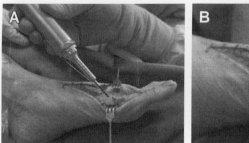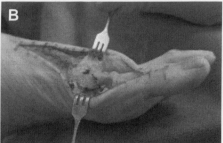

Fig. 2. (*A*) Placement of the Sonic Fusion pin for hallux valgus. After a drill hole is placed in the first metatarsal, the Sonic Fusion pin is inserted. (*B*) Placement of Sonic Fusion pin for hallux valgus. After the Sonic Fusion pin is inserted, an ultrasound charge is applied (*A*) and the PLDA material diffuses into the capital fragment and the bone is fixated. Any prominent PLDA may be removed from the dorsal aspect of the capital fragment and in this instance a hot cautery was used to melt the residual PLDA to sit flush dorsally.

The newer generation plate fixation devices allow the screw to lock into the plate, with the latest versions being anatomically constructed for the capital fragment osteotomies. These locking plates provide increased stability with only unicortical purchase because each screw locks into the plate to form a single construct. Locking plates have been described as an internal type of external fixator. Because they do not rely on friction to provide fixation, periosteal blood supply is better preserved, which may lead to better healing. However, locking plates add significant expense to the surgery and, as such, locking plates probably have limited indications in the fixation of capital metatarsal osteotomies (**Figs. 3** and **4**).

SONIC FUSION CASE PRESENTATION
Patient History

A 49-year-old patient with diabetes and peripheral neuropathy had a history of a bunion deformity and hallux hammertoe with a chronic ulcerations to the first metatarsophalangeal joint and plantar aspect of the hallux interphalangeal joint (IPJ) for many

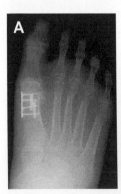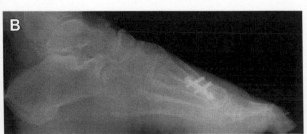

Fig. 3. (*A*) Postoperative radiographs of a foot following insertion of compression screws and locking plate in the correction of hallux valgus with limitus and arthritis. (*B*) The same patient as in (*A*). This patient had multiple cystic changes within the arthritic head. As a result, it was determined that a locking plate would be most beneficial to stabilize the osteotomy. This patient went on to successful healing of her surgery with no complications.

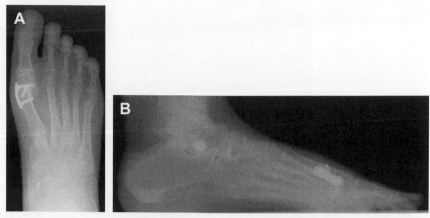

Fig. 4. (*A*) This patient presented with congenital pes planus, with posterior tibial dysfunction and a bunion. (*B*) The same patient as in (*A*). The patient underwent a Kidner procedure, TAL, subtalar arthroereisis, and bunionectomy. A chevron was chosen for the bunionectomy and the anatomic locking plate used allows for addition movement of the capital fragment while maintaining solid fixation. TAL, Tendo-achilles Lengthening.

years. The chosen procedure was to perform a hallux IPJ fusion with an Austin bunionectomy.

Physical Examination

The hallux had moderate abduction and valgus rotation. The patient had a mild dorsomedial bony prominence at the first metatarsophalangeal joint. The hallux IPJ was contracted plantarly and in valgus. There was decreased arch height bilaterally. The pedal pulses were palpable with capillary refill time between approximately 2 and 3 seconds. There was no pallor on elevation. The patient had diminished sensation to sharp/dull and light touch. Protective threshold was absent. The ulcer on the right hallux remained healed.

Imaging and Additional Testing

Preoperative radiographs revealed a first intermetatarsal angle of 12° and a hallux valgus angle of 36°. The metatarsal head showed moderate hypertrophy (**Fig. 5**). At 3-month follow-up, the radiographs revealed an intermetatarsal angle of 9° and a hallux valgus angle of 10° (See **Fig. 8**).

The Procedure

This case concerns the correction of hallux valgus using a SonicPin (Stryker, Mahwah NJ). The SonicPin is a copolymer of the dextro and levo stereoisomers of polylactic acid. The levo enantiomer makes a crystalline structure that is strong and has a lengthy resorption process. The dextro enantiomer has an amorphous structure that is weaker than Poly lactic acid levo anantomer (PLLA) and has a more rapid resorption process. Manipulation of the composition of the two monomers of the copolymer can adjust the strength and degradation profile. The blend of the Sonic Fusion pin seeks to achieve the greatest strength and degradation profile. This copolymer maintains its mechanical strength for at least 8 weeks and is fully resorbed within approximately 2 years.

The patient was brought into the operating room, a well-padded calf tourniquet was applied, and the limb was sterilely prepped and draped. Attention was directed

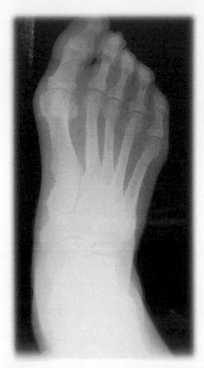

Fig. 5. Preoperative radiographs revealed a first intermetatarsal angle of 12° and a hallux valgus angle of 36°. The metatarsal head shows hypertrophy. A hallux hammertoe with significant hallux abductus interphalangeus is noted.

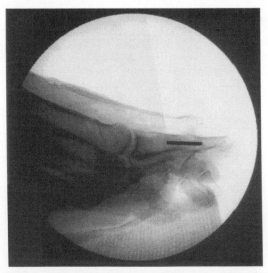

Fig. 6. Immediate postoperative films show excellent correction of the intermetatarsal angle and Hallux Abductovalgus angle.

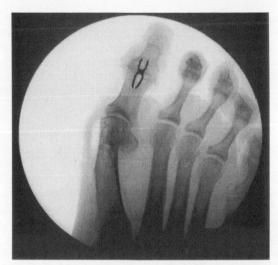

Fig. 7. The same patient as in **Fig. 6**. Note the radiolucent channels into which the absorbable pins are inserted. Note also the excellent bony apposition of the hallux IPJ fusion site.

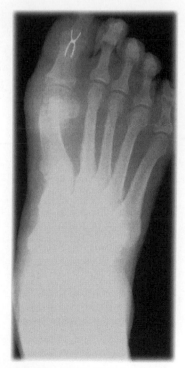

Fig. 8. At 3 months, the radiographs reveal an intermetatarsal angle of 9° and a hallux valgus angle of 10°. The SonicPin holes can be seen.

to the dorsomedial aspect of the patient's foot where a 6-cm longitudinal incision was made and a standard chevron cut was made into the first metatarsal after the medial eminence was removed. Once osteotomized, the head was shifted laterally and impacted on the proximal part of the metatarsal in its corrected position. Once in its corrected position, the osteotomy was stabilized using guidewires using care to ensure that the guidewire did not penetrate the plantar cortex. A guide hole was drilled, and a 26-mm SonicPin was inserted into each of the screw holes. The device was engaged and sonic energy caused the distal tip to semiliquefy and fill the medullary canal as the pin was inserted flush into the bone. A second pin was inserted in a similar fashion. The medial bone shelf was then removed.

At this time, attention was directed to the hallux IPJ. Using standard technique, an incision was made over the hallux IPJ and bone was resected distally and proximally An X-Fuse implant was inserted into the joint to provide fixation. At this time it was noted that the patient's preoperative deformity was corrected (**Figs. 6** and **7**) and the capsule and skin were closed in layers. The foot was dressed in dry sterile dressing and a well-padded posterior splint was applied.

After surgery, the patient was placed in a splint for 2 weeks, with heel-touch weight bearing because of the history of diabetes. After this, the patient was progressed into in a Cam boot. At 6 weeks after surgery, the patient was slowly transitioned to regular tennis shoes. The first intermetatarsal angle was measured at 9° and the hallux valgus angle was measured at 10° at 3 months after surgery (**Fig. 8**). At 6 months, the patient was well healed, back to full activity, with no recurrence of deformity and no complications associated with the resorbable fixation (**Fig. 9**).

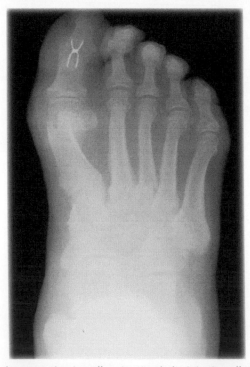

Fig. 9. At 6 months, the correction is well maintained, the joint is well aligned, and there are no complications appreciated with placement of the resorbable Sonic Fusion pins.

SUMMARY

First reported more than a century ago, capital osteotomies of the first metatarsal remain a tested method for the correction of hallux valgus. As the osteotomies have evolved, so too have the fixation options. Advancements in implant technology continue to provide new means of fixation. Some implants have been developed to help reduce operating time, such as self-drilling and self-tapping screws. Some implants have been developed to provide extra stabilization. However, the question must be asked: is the development going too far? Many capital osteotomies are inherently stable and rarely, if ever, require a costly locking plate. In contrast, other implants, such as absorbable implants, may be underused. This may be because of the complications of earlier generation implants that often caused inflammatory reactions. Newer bioabsorbable implants have a strength and degradation profile that provides adequate strength to support healing bone and to have minimal inflammation. Current research and development are leading to more cost-effective absorbable implants with greater ease of use for the treatment of hallux valgus.

REFERENCES

1. Nix S, Smith M, Vincenzino B. Prevalence of hallux valgus in the general population: a systematic review and metaanalysis. J Foot Ankle Res 2010;3:21.
2. Helal B. Surgery for adolescent hallux valgus. Clin Orthop 1981;157:50–63.
3. Reverdin J. De la deviation en dehors du gros orl (hallux valgus) et son traitement chirurgical. Trans Int Med Congress 1881;2:408–12.
4. Roux C. Aux pieds sensibles. Rev Med Suisse Romande 1920;40:62–5.
5. Snyder AJ, Hetherington VJ. Overview of distal first metatarsal osteotomies. In: Hetherington VJ, editor. Hallux valgus and forefoot surgery. New York: Churchill Livingstone; 1994. p. 163–7.
6. Hohmann G. Symptomatische oder physiologische behandlung des hallux valgus. Münch Med Wochenschr 1921;33:1042–5.
7. Hawkins FB, Mitchell CC, Hedrick DW. Correction of hallux valgus by metatarsal osteotomy. J Bone Joint Surg Am 1945;27(3):387–94.
8. Mitchell C, Fleming J, Allen R, et al. Osteotomy-bunionectomy for hallux valgus. J Bone Joint Surg Am 1958;40(1):41–60.
9. Wilson JN. Oblique displacement osteotomy for hallux valgus. J Bone Joint Surg Br 1963;45:552–6.
10. Austin DW, Leventon EO. Scientific exhibit of V-osteotomy of the first metatarsal head. Chicago: AAOS; 1968.
11. Austin DW, Leventon EO. A new osteotomy for hallux valgus: a horizontally directed "V" displacement osteotomy of the metatarsal head for hallux valgus and primus varus. Clin Orthop Relat Res 1981;157:25–30.
12. Johnson JB, Smith SB. Preliminary report on derotational angulational, transpositional osteotomy: a new approach to hallux abducto valgus surgery. J Am Podiatry Assoc 1974;64(8):667–75.
13. Hattrup SJ, Johnson KA. Chevron osteotomy: analysis of factors in patient's dissatisfaction. Foot Ankle 1985;5(6):327–32.
14. Feit EM, Scherer P, De Yoe B, et al. The nonfixated Austin bunionectomy: a retrospective study of one-hundred procedures. J Foot Ankle Surg 1997;36(5):347–52.
15. Gudas CJ. Compression screw fixation in proximal first metatarsal osteotomies for metatarsus primus varus: initial observations. J Foot Surg 1979;18(1):10–5.

16. Jahss MH, Troy AI, Kummer F. Roentgenographic and mathematical analysis of first metatarsal osteotomies for metatarsus primus varus: a comparative study. Foot Ankle 1985;5(6):280–321.
17. Calder JD, Holligdale JP, Pearse MF. Screw versus suture fixation of Mitchell's osteotomy: a prospective, randomised study. J Bone Joint Surg Br 1999;81(4): 621–4.
18. Bussewitz BW, Levar T, Hyer CF. Modern techniques in hallux abducto valgus surgery. Clin Podiatr Med Surg 2011;28:287–303.
19. Pelto-Vasenius K, Hirvensalo E, Vasenius J, et al. Osteolytic changes after polyglycolide pin fixation in chevron osteotomy. Foot Ankle Int 1997;18:21–5.
20. Barca F, Busa R. Austin/Chevron osteotomy fixed with bioabsorbable poly-L-lactic acid single screw. J Foot Ankle Surg 1997;36:15–20.
21. Hirvensalo E, Böstman O, Törmälä P, et al. Chevron osteotomy fixed with absorbable polyglycolide pins. Foot Ankle 1991;11:212–8.
22. Small HN, Braly WG, Tullos HS. Fixation of the Chevron osteotomy utilizing absorbable polydioxanon pins. Foot Ankle Int 1995;16:346–50.
23. Winemaker MJ, Amendola A. Comparison of bioabsorbable pins and Kirschner wires in the fixation of chevron osteotomies for hallux valgus. Foot Ankle Int 1996;17:623–8.
24. Gill LH, Martin DF, Coumas JM, et al. Fixation with bioabsorbable pins in chevron bunionectomy. J Bone Joint Surg Am 1997;79:1510–8.
25. Alcelik I, Alnaib M, Pollock R, et al. Bioabsorbable fixation for Mitchell's bunionectomy osteotomy. J Foot Ankle Surg 2009;48:9–14.
26. Caminear DS, Pavlovich R Jr, Peitrzak WS. Fixation of the chevron osteotomy with an absorbable copolymer pin for treatment of hallux valgus deformity. J Foot Ankle Surg 2005;44:203–10.
27. DeOrio JK, Ware AW. Single absorbable polydioxanone pin fixation for distal chevron bunion osteotomies. Foot Ankle Int 2001;22:832–5.
28. Abdulazim A, Penzkofer R, Wipf F, et al. Paper 28: Ultrasonic welding of bioabsorbable pins in cancellous bone for fracture fixation. J Bone Joint Surg Br 2011;92(Suppl I):75.
29. Meara DJ, Knoll MR, Holmes JD, et al. Fixation of Le Fort I osteotomies with poly-DL-lactic acid mesh and ultrasonic welding – A new technique. J Oral Maxillofac Surg 2012;70(5):1139–44.
30. Buijs GJ, van der Houwen EB, Stegenga B, et al. Mechanical strength and stiffness of the biodegradable SonicWeld Rx osteofixation system. J Oral Maxillofac Surg 2009;67(4):782–7.
31. Heiss C, Alt V, Robioneck B, et al. Sonic Fusion Technologie zur Verankerung von Polymerimplanten im Knochen – Tierexperimentelle Untersuchungen am Osteotomiemodell. Meeting Abstract. Deutscher Kongress für Orthopädie und Unfallchirurgie, 75. Jahrestagung der Deutschen Gesellschaft für Unfallchirurgie, 97. Tagung der Deutschen Gesellschaft für Orthopädie und Orthopädische Chirurgie, 52. Tagung des Berufsverbandes der Fachärzte für Orthopädie und Unfallchirurgie. Berlin, 25-28.10.2011. Düsseldorf: German Medical Science GMS Publishing House; 2011.
32. Schneider M, Loukota R, Reitmeier B, et al. Bone block fixation by ultrasound activated resorbable pin osteosynthesis: a biomechanical in vitro analysis of stability. Oral Surg Oral Med Oral Pathol Oral Radiol Endod 2010;109(1):79–85.
33. Sammarco VJ, Acevedo J. Stability and fixation techniques in first metatarsal osteotomies. Foot Ankle Clin 2001;6(3):409–31.

Opening Base Wedge Osteotomies in Hallux Valgus Correction
Are Anatomic Plates the Answer?

Brian S. Stover, DPM

KEYWORDS

- Opening base wedge osteotomy • Hallux valgus • Bunionectomy • First metatarsal
- Arthrex POW plate

KEY POINTS

- Opening base wedge osteotomies can provide adequate reduction of large IM angles with predictable results utilizing anatomic locking plates.
- Opening base wedge osteotomies can provide reduction of HAV deformities without shortening of the first metatarsal that can be seen with other procedures.
- Anatomic locking plates can provide a rigid construct for an osteotomy to decrease risk of nonunion.

There are more than 100 procedures described for the surgical correction of a hallux abducto valgus (HAV) deformity. Procedures range from capsulotendon balancing to head or basilar osteotomies and even double osteotomies of the first metatarsal.[1] Many of these procedures have failed to gain popularity because of technical difficulty, high complication rates, and lack of appropriate and/or stable fixation methods. There are a few procedures that have stood the test of time and have even become easier to perform because of advances in fixation techniques and materials. An example of this would be the lapidus arthrodesis for a large first-second intermetatarsal angle (IMA). The lapidus over the years has become more favorable because of better fixation, even for those physicians who were intimidated by the procedure. There are still those who avoid the lapidus because of concerns of fusing a "normal" joint or needing a patient to remain non–weight bearing for an extended period of time. Even though there are many advocating early weight bearing with a lapidus,[2] many physicians are still fearful of a resultant nonunion or malunion secondary to early weight bearing.

It is for this reason that a need still exists for a stable, proximal procedure capable of reducing a large IMA without significant shortening of the first ray. The opening base

Funding Sources: None reported.
Conflict of Interest: None reported.
Southeastern Sports Medicine, 21 Turtle Creek, Asheville, NC 28803, USA
E-mail address: stover.brian@gmail.com

wedge osteotomy (OBWO) was first introduced in 1923 by Trethowan. He described it as a procedure for the correction of severe HAV in the juvenile or adolescent patient.[3] He further described the procedure as leaving the lateral cortex intact. In 1983, Beronio writes about maintaining the opening wedge with the resected medial eminence.[4] This procedure has fallen out of favor because of the need for bone graft, lack of stable fixation, fear of jamming the joint, prolonged period of non–weight bearing, and concerns of delayed or nonunions.

New plating systems may provide a solution for many of these concerns and resuscitate a procedure that is nearly extinct. The Arthrex Opening Wedge Low Profile Plate and Screw System (LPS) (Arthrex Inc., Naples, FL) allows surgeons to gain comfort in performing the OBWO because of the incorporated central spacer. The variable-sized spacers allow for "dialing in" of the correction and maintain the opening of the osteotomy. This plating system provides stable fixation and nearly nullifies the need for bone graft. Among surgeons, the concern of weight bearing in a patient still exists, even with this plating system. The next generation of this plate is the Proximal Opening Wedge (POW) plate. The design has moved from the familiar L-shape of the LPS plate to a T-shaped design more consistent with the tibial opening wedge plates (**Figs. 1–3**). In addition to a design change, this plate offers locking screws, which allows for a much more rigid construct that will afford earlier weight bearing.

SURGICAL TECHNIQUE

With the patient secured to the table in a supine position, hemostasis is obtained with a calf or thigh tourniquet. An incision is made extending from the base of the proximal phalanx to the first metatarsocuneiform joint. Dissection is carried down to the metatarsal. A lateral release is performed distally with resection of the medial eminence. The medial eminence may be placed in saline for later use. Proximally, at a point 1.0 to 1.5 cm distal to the metatarsocuneiform joint, a 0.062-inch Kirschner wire is driven from dorsal to plantar into the lateral aspect of the metatarsal so as to protect the lateral hinge of the osteotomy from being broken. Care should be taken to verify that the wire is driven perpendicular to the weight-bearing surface as opposed to the metatarsal itself. This is to avoid any elevatus of the metatarsal. The periosteum is then lifted on the medial aspect of the metatarsal where the cut is to be made. At this point, a sagittal saw is used to make a single transverse osteotomy medial to lateral, parallel with the already placed guide wire. Again, care is needed not to breach

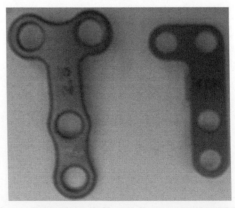

Fig. 1. Comparison of new POW plate (*left*) and first-generation LPS plate (*right*).

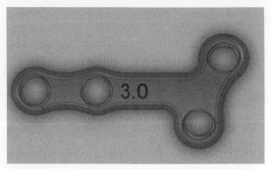

Fig. 2. Arthrex POW plate.

the lateral cortex. Once the osteotomy is completed, the wire is removed and can be placed into the medial aspect of the metatarsal head. One can now use this to lever the osteotomy open by pushing or pulling the Kirschner wire distally. It may be necessary to introduce a 10-mm osteotome or mini-lamina spreader to pry the osteotomy open. At this time, the wedge portion of the POW plate can be introduced into the osteotomy. Fluoroscopy is used to verify translocation of the metatarsal head over sesamoids and reduction of IMA. A 3-mm or 4-mm wedge is usually appropriate. Once satisfied with correction, screw placement can commence. This author's preference is starting with the most proximal distal screw, placing a nonlocking screw first to get the plate in good contact with the bone. This is then followed with locking screws in the remaining holes (**Figs. 4** and **5**). The previously placed nonlocking screw can then be swapped out for a locking variety of appropriate length. All screws should be bicortical, and this can be verified with fluoroscopy.

At this point, the remaining gap can be filled in with either the crushed eminence that was saved, cancellous bone chips, or other bone void filler of the surgeon's preference. Finally, evaluation of range of motion and position of the hallux is done, and

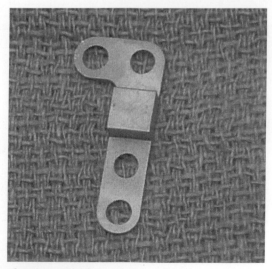

Fig. 3. Wedge side of Arthrex LPS plate.

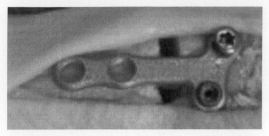

Fig. 4. Placement of nonlocking (dorsal) and locking screws (plantar).

any further procedures can then be performed. Layered closure followed by a compression dressing finishes the procedure (**Fig. 6**).

DISCUSSION

Since the inception of the OBWO, there has been significant resistance and debate surrounding perceived complications or downfalls of the procedure. Of these, the need for bone graft, lack of stable fixation, fear of jamming the joint, prolonged period of non–weight bearing, and concerns of delayed or nonunions are the most common stated. With the use of an anatomic wedge plate, the need for harvesting a graft of sufficient size and strength is no longer a valid concern. The plates are designed with varying wedge sizes to correct a varying degree of intermetatarsal angles with numerous manufacturers having similar plate designs, both locking and nonlocking. The POW plate, in particular, ranges in wedge sizes from a 2 mm up to a 7 mm. A study using the LPS plate from Arthrex demonstrated that the mean correction with these plates was 3° for every millimeter wedge.[5] Therefore, even the most severe of HAV deformities may be adequately treated with a wedge plate.

A major concern in performing any HAV correction is shortening of the first metatarsal and disrupting the parabolic relationship of the lesser metatarsals. If too much shortening is to occur, concern arises about lesser metatarsal overload, resulting in

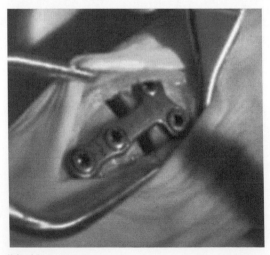

Fig. 5. Plate with all locking screws.

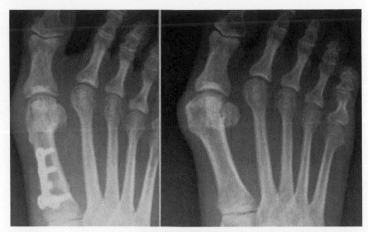

Fig. 6. Preoperative (*right*) and postoperative (*left*) radiographs of POW plate for opening base wedge osteotomy.

pain, calluses, or stress fracture. The OBWO is one of the only HAV procedures that inherently avoids shortening of the metatarsal. There has been concern presented that the use of this procedure may in fact cause too much metatarsal lengthening, resulting in stiffness or jamming of the first metatarsophalangeal joint. Budny and colleagues,[6] in a bench study, found that the average increase in metatarsal length was 1% to 3% of original metatarsal length. This study was performed on sawbone models. In vitro studies using low-profile plating systems have demonstrated lengthening of the first metatarsal or metatarsal protrusion distance to be 2.3 and 2.6 mm, respectively. In the first study, in which the procedure was performed on 64 feet, an average increase in metatarsal length of 2.3 mm was not significant enough for the occurrence of transfer metatarsalgia.[7] Another study of 18 procedures confirmed the absence of transfer metatarsalgia. In fact, it advocated for the use of a low-profile opening wedge plate in cases with a short metatarsal or prior failed correction.[8]

Nonunions and delayed unions are an inherent complication in any osteotomy. There is speculation that with the OBWO, the use of graft and instability are the reasons for nonunion. What is now known is that a rigid construct decreases risk of nonunion. Prior attempts at fixation for OBWO, including staples, wires, cerclage wire, and no fixation have all been reported. Most recent studies using an anatomic plate with spacer have shown very low nonunion rates. In fact, one study using locking screws, similar to those found in the POW plate, suggested a 0% nonunion rate. It is important to note that in the study delayed unions and nonunions did occur in a subgroup using a plating system with nonlocking screws. Another point in this was the lack of dorsal malunion, as the plate rigidly prevents shear and bending moments.[9] It reportedly takes 5.9 weeks to see fusion with the use of an anatomic plate of this type.[5] Of course, appropriate patient and procedure selection are always most important in avoiding any complication.

Weight-bearing status has been another suggested reason to avoid this procedure. With the use of locking plates, surgeons have been pushing the limits of earlier ambulation. Of the studies reviewed for this article, almost all allowed some form of weight bearing either immediately or 2 weeks after surgery. Using locking plates, confidence in successful outcome is improved even with early weight bearing. Most patients are back to normal shoe gear at about 6 weeks. This is fairly consistent with what is seen with other HAV procedures.

SUMMARY

Most surgeons have a preferred or favorite procedure when it comes to correction of HAV. With the advances in technology, we should constantly reassess the value of a procedure. We should strive to understand the indications and limitations of the procedures we choose. Understanding that with the improvement in hardware, procedures that were once thought to be irrelevant can provide the correction that we want with the reliability that we need. The OBWO has had its shortcomings in the past. Anatomic plates are the answer to these shortcomings and provide for stable, predictable correction with few complications, affording early weight bearing.

REFERENCES

1. Pinney S, Song K, Chou L. Surgical treatment of severe hallux valgus: the state of practice among academic foot and ankle surgeons. Foot Ankle Int 2006;27(11): 970–3.
2. Blitz NM. Emerging concepts with post-lapidus bunionectomy weightbearing. Podiatry Today 2012;25(9):58. Available at: http://www.podiatrytoday.com/emerging-concepts-post-lapidus-bunionectomy-weightbearing. Accessed September 6, 2012.
3. Amarnek D, Juda E, Oloff L, et al. Opening base wedge of the first metatarsal utilizing rigid external fixation. J Foot Surg 1986;25(4):321–6.
4. Beronio JP. One approach to a viable method of obtaining cancellous bone for grafting. J Foot Surg 1983;22:240–2.
5. Shurnas P, Watson T, Crislip T. Proximal first metatarsal opening wedge osteotomy with a low profile plate. Foot Ankle Int 2009;30(9):865–72.
6. Budny A, Masadeh S, Lyons M II, et al. The opening base wedge osteotomy and subsequent lengthening of the first metatarsal: an in vitro study. J Foot Ankle Surg 2009;48(6):662–7.
7. Nikiforos P. Proximal opening-wedge osteotomy of the first metatarsal for hallux valgus using a low profile plate. Foot Ankle Int 2009;30(10):976–80.
8. Wukich D, Roussel A, Dial D. Correction of metatarsus primus varus with an opening wedge plate: a review of 18 procedures. J Foot Ankle Surg 2009;48(4):420–6.
9. Smith B, Hyer C, DeCarbo W, et al. Opening wedge osteotomies for correction of hallux valgus: a review of wedge plate fixation. Foot Ankle Spec 2009;2(6): 277–82.

Second Metatarsophalangeal Joint Pathology and Freiberg Disease

Amber Shane, DPM[a],*, Christopher Reeves, DPM[b],
Garrett Wobst, DPM[c], Paul Thurston, DPM[c]

KEYWORDS

- Predislocation syndrome • Plantar plate rupture • Crossover second toe
- Instability second toe • Freiberg disease • Freiberg infraction

KEY POINTS

- Second MTPJ pathology is a common and difficult problem with challenging treatment options for the Foot and Ankle Surgeon.
- Early recognition and stringent conservative treatment is paramount in treating these chronic and progressive disorders, however surgical treatment may ultimately be unavoidable for these patients.
- Recent advancements in surgical techniques have been outlined and show reproducible results for the treatment of second MTPJ pathology.

ANATOMY

First we must discuss the dysfunctional second metatarsophalangeal joint (MTPJ) when evaluating the functional anatomy of the joint. The second MTPJ has a number of unique factors that may predispose the joint to pathology. Many intrinsic and extrinsic structures cross the joint and each play a biomechanical role in function. An in-depth anatomic evaluation of the second MTPJ is beyond the scope of this review; however, basic understanding of the structure and forces that cross the joint is necessary.

The lesser MTPJs are crossed dorsally by 2 extensor tendons, the longus and brevis. The extensor digitorum brevis joins the longus on the fibular side of the digit and blends with the longus to cross the MTJP. The tendons act to dorsiflex the digits during the swing phase of gait, and stabilize the digits during propulsion.[1] The sheath of the extensor tendons blend with the capsule of the MTPJ, which subsequently

[a] Orlando Foot and Ankle Clinics, 250 North Alafaya Trail, Suite 105, Orlando, FL 32825, USA;
[b] Orlando Foot and Ankle Clinics, 2111 Glenwood Drive, Suite 104, Winter Park, FL 32792, USA;
[c] PGY-3, Florida Hospital East Orlando, 7975 Lake Underhill Road, Suite 210, Orlando, FL 32822, USA
* Corresponding author.
E-mail address: ashane@orlandofootandankle.com

Clin Podiatr Med Surg 30 (2013) 313–325
http://dx.doi.org/10.1016/j.cpm.2013.04.009   **podiatric.theclinics.com**
0891-8422/13/$ – see front matter © 2013 Elsevier Inc. All rights reserved.

attaches to the plantar structures, including the plantar plate and deep transverse ligament.[2] This anatomic configuration allows for a strong dorsiflexory attitude of the proximal phalanx, which may explain the dorsal dislocation of the proximal phalanx on the metatarsal head often seen with pathology of this joint. In contrast, the flexor tendons function as the primary flexors of the interphalangeal joints, with a passive plantarflexory force across the MTPJ.[2]

A unique aspect of the second MTPJ is that it has 2 dorsal interosseous muscles crossing the joint. The remaining lesser digits have both plantar and dorsal interosseous muscles. These interossei muscles serve to stabilize the MTPJ in the transverse plane.[2] Also unique to the second MTPJ is that the long flexor sits directly below the head of the metatarsal, rather than a slightly offset medial position, as noted on the other lesser rays.[3] This is thought to be a contributing factor to the painful synovitis often associated with pathology of the second MTPJ.

The lumbricals of the foot originate on the medial aspect of the long flexor tendons and attach on the medial aspect of the MTPJ capsule. This allows an unopposed adductory force across the MTPJ.[2] However, with an intact lateral capsule, plantar plate, and lateral collateral ligaments, this adductory force is easily balanced.[3]

A major structure of the second MTPJ is the plantar plate. The plate is a fibrocartilagenous structure, mainly composed of type I collagen and blended tissue elements from its attachments.[1,2] These attachments are extensive and include the deep transverse intermetatarsal ligament, plantar fascia, capsular tissues, interossei tendons, and flexor sheath. The plantar plate has been indicated as the major stabilizing structure of the second MTPJ.[1–8] It has a firm attachment to the base of the proximal phalanx, and to the collateral ligaments and plantar fascia; however, it has a weak fibrous attachment to the metatarsal neck.[1,6] Its primary functions are twofold: first, it resists tensile loads in the longitudinal direction, particularly when the second MTPJ is dorsiflexed; second, it provides cushioning to joint during weight bearing.[1,6] In conjunction with the interossei muscle, the plantar plate is the primary stabilizer of the second MTPJ in the transverse and sagittal planes.

PATHOLOGY

Pain while ambulating to the plantar aspect of the second MTPJ is a common occurrence seen by the foot and ankle specialist. Isolated second MTPJ pathology is rare, and is often associated with structural or biomechanical dysfunction of the foot. Typical associated conditions include hallux valgus deformity coupled with a hypermobile first ray, which creates an overloading syndrome to the second metatarsal head during propulsion. A pronated foot type overloading the medial column structures may also lead to second MTPJ dysfunction. Finally, ankle equinus must be evaluated, as a tight heel cord has been shown to increase forefoot pressures, which can play a role in the development of second MTPJ symptoms.

Numerous etiologies have been described in the literature, with much overlap of the accepted terminology. These include trauma, predislocation syndrome, overuse injury, stress fracture, avascular necrosis, capsulitis, synovitis, and systemic and isolated inflammatory conditions. Perhaps the most common of these conditions includes predislocation syndrome and avascular necrosis of the metatarsal head.

PREDISLOCATION SYNDROME

Predislocation syndrome was formally introduced by Yu and Judge in 1995 and again in their hallmark study in 2002.[9,10] However, with regard to pathology about the second MTPJ, numerous terms have been used to describe similar conditions concerning derangement of the joint. Miller published an extensive list of the terms that have been used to describe this condition; these include the following:

- Submetatarsal 2 syndrome
- Chronic lesser MTPJ dislocation
- Floating toe syndrome
- Lesser MTPJ instability syndrome
- Second MTPJ dislocation
- Crossover second-toe deformity
- Monoarticular nontraumatic synovitis

Predislocation has been described in any of the lesser rays; however, the second MTPJ is the most common of the joints involved. It has been described as a continuum of pathologic entities progressing from acute capsulitis to subacute plantar plate rupture and chronic dislocation of the joint.[2,9] The condition is progressive, with each stage weakening anatomic structures about the MTPJ, producing the next clinical signs and symptoms.

Etiology

There have been many causes suggested for the development of predislocation syndrome. These include hallux valgus deformity; hypermobile first ray; abnormal metatarsal parabola; traumatic, neuromuscular, anomalous muscle, and other anatomic abnormalities; and congenital causes.[11] Each of these causes hold merit on the development of the deformity; however, congenital predilection, combined with the aging process, female gender, and chronic ill-fitting shoe gear, may be the most likely cause.[9,11,12] Yu and colleagues[9] postulated that the common anatomic and biomechanical variants were the fundamental causes of the syndrome. They postulated that the long second metatarsal or pronated foot type created an increased plantar pressure to the second MTPJ, causing the progression of the disease.[9] However, there has been no consistent correlation between these biomechanical findings and predislocation syndrome in the literature. Kaz and Coughlin[12] radiographically examined 169 consecutive patients diagnosed with predislocation syndrome and found no statistical correlation between second metatarsal length, hallux valgus angle, Meary angle, or intermetatarsal angle, dispelling the notion that common structural abnormalities are the root cause of the deformity. Several investigators suggest that use of high-heeled shoes and tight toe box increasing the forefoot pressure may predispose individuals to lesser metatarsalgia.[9,11,12]

As mentioned previously, women appear to have a preponderance to the deformity. This is likely because of the aforementioned high-fashion shoe gear that tends to be associated with the syndrome. Age is another factor that appears to be associated with the condition. In the series by Kaz and Coughlin,[12] of 169 patients radiographically examined, 146 (86%) of these were women. This is similar to other reports in which most subjects are women, ranging from 70% to 100%.[2,3,11–18]

Clinical Presentation

Predislocation syndrome typically begins as a subtle vague complaint of pain and inflammation of the plantar aspect of the second MTPJ while the patient is ambulating. Yu and Judge[10] described a "pain out of proportion" scenario with respect to the initial clinical presentation. Early in the clinical presentation, no deformity, crepitus, or malalignment is noted.[2] There may be a subtle deviation noted between the second and third metatarsals, leading to the improper diagnosis of intermetatarsal neuroma of the second interspace.[3,12–16] However, this condition rarely elicits complaints of numbness, burning, or sharp shooting pain into the adjacent digits, typically associated with the clinical presentation of neuroma. Often the patient complains of severe pain while walking barefoot.[9] The patient may also subjectively describe the feeling of walking on a "stone" or a "lump in their sock."[9]

As the deformity progresses, the digit tends to become elevated, and may progress to the proximal phalanx, dorsally dislocating on the second metatarsal head.[12,13] Typically the patient will complain that it feels as if the digit is "trying to dislocate" or "go out of position."[9] The second digit loses purchase with the ground, and a positive vertical stress test is noted (**Fig. 1**). Radiographs echo the clinical presentation, displaying medial and dorsal deviation of the second MTPJ.

This final stage of the disease lends itself to the term "crossover second digit," because the second digit is dorsally and medially dislocated over the hallux. At this stage, dermatologic lesions are typically present on the dorsal aspect of the proximal interphalangeal joint because of pressure in shoe gear (**Fig. 2**).

Staging

Yu and Judge[10] proposed a classification scheme based on clinical and radiographic findings at the time of presentation (**Table 1**). It is worth noting that predislocation syndrome is a chronic problem developing over an extended period of time, and that the stages described are a continuum of these symptoms. Often one stage can blend into the next with multiple aspects of both stages.

In stage 1, no malalignment is noted. There is typically palpable thickness or frank edema plantarly about the second MTPJ. Tenderness is noted at the extreme ends of range or motion exercises. In stage 2, there is noticeable malalignment both clinically and radiographically. Loss of toe purchase is noted when weight bearing. Edema is noted both plantarly and often dorsally. In stage 3, the deviation is significantly more pronounced with subluxation or dislocation likely. Often this is where the crossover second toe deformity is noted. Edema extends into the digit (**Fig. 3**).

Sferra and Arndt[11] described an alternative staging system incorporating the pathonomonic positive vertical stress test to help stage the disease (**Table 2**). In grade 0, there is subjective joint pain and swelling without joint instability or deviation, and a negative vertical stress test. Grade 1 is characterized by a positive vertical stress test, without joint deformity. Grade 2 has a positive stress test with notable joint malalignment. Grade 3 is characterized by a flexible or partially reducible dislocated joint, whereas grade 4 is a dislocated joint that is nonreducible.

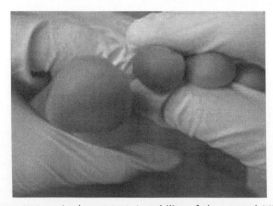

Fig. 1. Vertical stress test, or Lachman test. Instability of the second MTPJ is defined as a 5-mm translation of the joint. Pain is typically reproducible during this test.

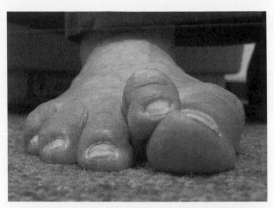

Fig. 2. Clinical picture of end-stage predislocation syndrome. Note the crossover digit of the second on the hallux.

Conservative Treatment

Typical conservative treatment modalities are aimed at stopping the progression of the disease with relief of painful symptoms. The multimodal approach seems to have the most benefit with a combination of pharmacologic and splintage treatments. Initially, shoe gear modification, including wide toe box, reduction of heel height, and rocker bottom–type sole, may alleviate early symptomatology. Oral anti-inflammatory medications, including corticosteroids and nonsteroidal anti-inflammatory drugs, are a mainstay treatment for managing this disorder. Pharmacologic treatment in combination with plantarflexory toe taping, metatarsal pads, or commercially available toe splints may offload and stabilize this joint, reducing advancement of the syndrome. However, an astute practitioner must educate patients that these modalities may not completely stop the progression of the disorder.

Intra-articular cortical steroid injections have been proposed as a possible nonsurgical treatment, and many reports have commented on using this modality in the treatment of the disease. The use of intra-articular steroid injections for predislocation syndrome is controversial, with many investigators advising against this practice. The adverse effects of periarticular steroid injections has been noted in the literature, namely the weakening of the stabilizing soft tissue structures about the joint. Reis and

Table 1
Stages of predislocation syndrome

Stage	Clinical Presentation	Radiographic Presentation
1	• Subtle, mild edema • Plantar thickness • Pain out of proportion • No malalignment • Pain at end of range of motion	• No change
2	• Loss of toe purchase • Notable deviation of digit • Increased edema about joint	• Deviation of digit noted • Subluxation is often seen
3	• Pronounced edema extending into digit • "Crossover" digit typically seen.	• Dorsal dislocation • Severe deviation of digit

From Yu GV, Judge MS, Hudson JR, et al. Predislocation syndrome: progressive subluxation/dislocation of the lesser metatarsophalangeal joint. J Am Podiatr Med Assoc 2002;92(2):182–99.

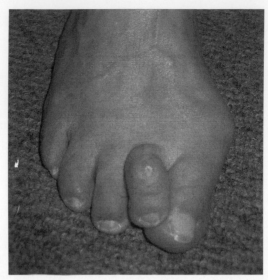

Fig. 3. Predislocation syndrome.

colleagues[19] were the first to report frank dislocation of the second MTPJ after local steroid injection into this area for treatment of stage 1 predislocation syndrome. Other studies[20] have demonstrated significant destruction of fibrocytes and decreased tensile strength into the ligamentous structure about the joint after a single injection of corticosteroid.

Surgical Treatments

The conservative measures listed previously are often sufficient to provide pain relief, and lessening the progression of the disease. Often, however, these modalities are not successful with advanced disease, and surgical intervention is warranted. An array of surgical procedures has been described for treatment of predislocation syndrome. Typically the focus of surgical treatment consists of soft tissue releases and tendon transfers to realign the deranged joint. Synovectomy, ligament release, and lumbrical tendon release have been well represented in the literature. Tendon transfers, such as extensor digitorum brevis re-routing, first described by Haddad and colleagues,[21] noted satisfactory results in 68% of subjects. They re-routed the EDB inferior to the deep transverse intermetatarsal ligament to reduce a dorsal dislocated joint. Barca and Acciaro[22] reported a technique using a Girdlestone-Taylor–type tendon transfer,

Table 2
Staging of predislocation syndrome using the vertical stress test

Stage	Vertical Stress Test	Clinical Presentation
0	• Negative	• Subjective joint pain
1	• Positive	• No deformity
2	• Positive	• Notable joint malalignment
3	• Positive	• Flexible/Reducible deformity
4	• Positive	• Nonreducible deformity

Adapted from Sferra J, Arndt S. The crossover toe and valgus toe deformity. Foot Ankle Clin 2011;16(4):609–20.

with medial capsule release, with 83% of subjects reporting good to excellent results at follow-up. The addition of a distal metatarsal osteotomy improved these outcomes, with decompression of the affected joint, and ease of realignment. However, these studies all reported a percentage of subjects with recurrent symptoms and some degree of return of initial deformity.

Recently, the focus of the disease has been on the repair of the fundamental deforming factor, the plantar plate, and realignment of the deranged joint. Early reports highlighted a separate plantar approach for primary repair of the plantar plate, with or without adjunctive osteotomy and soft tissue procedures. Powless and Elze[23] looked at 58 patients with diagnosed predislocation syndrome, and underwent a primary repair using a plantar approach, with 56 patients reporting symptom relief. Although this series reported good results with the technique, plantar incisions, particularly about the weight-bearing areas on the foot, are frequently noted with complications. A newer technique, described by Weil and colleagues[24] and again by Coughlin and colleagues,[25] outlined a dorsal approach, combining soft tissue releases, distal metatarsal osteotomy, and primary repair of the plantar plate. Weil and colleagues[24] examined 15 cases, with an average follow-up of 22 months; 77% of the patients had satisfactory results.[24] Gregg and colleagues[26] performed a similar case series of 35 cases with similar good to excellent results.

Although many surgical treatments have been reported, the evidence appears to be in favor of a combination of tissue balancing, repair, and decompression osteotomy for lasting treatment of this complex deformity.

FREIBERG DISEASE

Freiberg brought osteonecrosis of the second metatarsal head to light in 1914.[27] Freiberg disease, although uncommon, should be in the differential diagnosis of second MTPJ pathology. Its presentation is predominantly in the adolescent female population of ages 11 to 17,[28] is unilateral, and presents as pain to the second and sometimes third MTPJ. Limited range of motion, pain when weight bearing relieved with rest, and localized swelling to the joint in clinical examination are common findings as well.

Etiology

Vascular compromise and trauma are agreed on theories of its cause. Anatomic studies conducted have shown evidence of vascular variations, as well as absence of normal arterial flow to the affected metatarsal, rendering the blood flow to collateral circulation. Traumatic theory applies to biomechanical alterations, such as an elongated second metatarsal enduring stress (**Fig. 4**). Structural deformities, such as hallux valgus or hallux rigidus, are culprits as well, which can transfer the weight lateral to the second metatarsal. With this increased stress through gait, micro trauma to the head of the metatarsal may occur. Systemic disease must also be considered. Diseases, such as systemic lupus erythematosus, and any disease that causes a hypercoagulable state, can lead to Freiberg disease. Early recognition, although difficult to diagnose in many instances, can lead to less aggressive treatment and favorable outcomes, as the early stages usually respond to conservative treatment more effectively.

Clinical Presentation

As mentioned, Freiberg disease usually presents in the adolescent female population as forefoot pain localized most commonly to the second MTPJ. It may present with

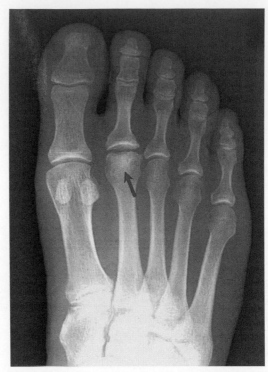

Fig. 4. Traumatic theory of Freiberg disease of the second MTPJ. A long second metatarsal is often noted radiographically causing increased pressure to the metatarsal head. The arrow indicates the erosion of the subchondral plate and regression of the metatarsal head, leading to severe joint destruction.

pain during weight bearing, pain and limited range of motion, and clinical evidence of swelling to the joint. Radiographs are used to discern the degree of damage. Early stages of disease may not appear on standard radiographs, and advanced imaging, such as magnetic resonance imaging (MRI), may be useful. Early stages of damage on MRI will show increased signal intensity on T2 and short T1 inversion recovery, but as the disease becomes chronic, low signal intensity to the metatarsal head appears on T1 (**Fig. 5**).[29] In later stages of disease, standard radiographs with clinical symptoms present allow for a more rapid diagnosis. In the advanced stage, notable derangement and flattening of the metatarsal head and periarticular area with loose bodies can be appreciated (**Fig. 6**).

Staging

Freiberg first described a classification scheme in his landmark article in 1914.[27] His classification scheme was established from a combination of radiographic, clinical, and suggested surgical findings of 6 female subjects with similar presenting syndromes (**Table 3**). Although widely used, the Freiberg classification system has been adapted, and classification schemes now help direct the treatment protocols for patients with this condition. The well-established classification proposed by Smillie[30] provides a systematic diagnostic and treatment plan (**Table 4**).

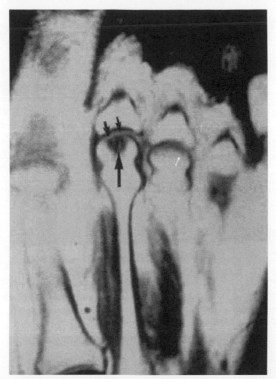

Fig. 5. Note the hypointense signal on the second metatarsal head (*arrow*) reflecting avascular disease and chronic edema.

Conservative Treatments

Conservative measures are typically used in early treatment. These measures consist of offloading the metatarsal through orthotics, metatarsal pads, modified shoe gear, and removable walking boots. If conservative measures fail, surgical options must be visited.

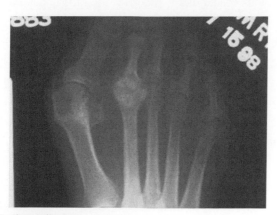

Fig. 6. End-stage Freiberg disease.

Table 3
Classification of Freiberg infraction, as described by Freiberg in 1914

Stage	Findings
1	• Articular cartilage intact • No degenerative disease
2	• Articular cartilage intact • Mild degenerative disease • Periarticular spurring
3	• Articular cartilage lost • Severe degenerative disease
4	• Epiphyseal dysplasia • Multiple joint involvement

Surgical Treatments

There are many surgical options, ranging from joint destructive to joint preserving. Smillie[30] first recommended operating on stages I, II, and III in an attempt to restore a new blood supply. A 14 × 5-mm slot is cut in the dorsum of the shaft of the metatarsal to gain access to the fracture site. The sclerotic borders are derided and roughened. The epiphyseal plate is the fenestrated. Postoperatively, the patient is placed in a cast for 12 weeks, then allowed to partial weight bear in a shoe.

Since Smillie's[30] original classification and treatment plan, many variations have evolved. El-Tayeby[31] demonstrated positive results with an interposition arthroplasty of the extensor digitorum longus acting as a spacer in the MTPJ. The extensor digitorum longus was cut 5 cm proximal to the joint. After the head of the metatarsal was remodeled, the extensor digitorum longus was sutured to the plantar plate and the most proximal segment was resutured to the periosteum of the metatarsal shaft. With this procedure, 7 of 13 patients had complete pain relief, 3 patients had mild pain relief, and 3 patients had moderate pain relief. Ten of the 13 had improved level of activity and 11 of the 13 had painless range of motion.

Metatarsal osteotomies are also used to dorsiflex the metatarsal head to allow for better articulation of the joint surfaces. These are typically reserved for later stage IV and V disease. Gauthier and Elbaz[32] brought this to the forefront with their dorsiflexory wedge osteotomy. The Weil osteotomy has also been used with many variations. Edmonson and colleagues[33] modified the traditional Weil osteotomy by

Table 4
Classification of Freiberg disease

Stage	Findings	Radiographic Presentation
1	• Fissure fracture	• No change
2	• Absorption of bone at metatarsal head • Fissuring of cartilage	• Sunken central metatarsal head
3	• Destruction of cartilage • Plantar metatarsal head viable	• Periarticular spurring • Entire metatarsal head appears sunken
4	• Entire metatarsal head avascular and nonviable, including plantar surface	• Loose bodies noted • Metatarsal head fractures noted
5	• Further destruction of metatarsal head	• Flattening of metatarsal head

From Smillie IS. Treatment of Freiberg's infraction. Proc R Soc Med 1967;60:29–31.

angling the apex of the osteotomy more proximal, which allowed the base of the wedge to encompass more diseased bone and allowing for easier fixation. Their study of 17 patients revealed a mean preoperative American Orthopaedic Foot and Ankle Society score of 51.6 (range 5–87) and a mean postoperative score of 87.6 (range 37–100), with all patients improving from their preoperative score.

Osteochondral autograft has been used with good success. Devries and colleagues[34] demonstrated successful results in the case of a 15-year-old with second metatarsal Freiberg disease who underwent an Osteochondral Autograft Transplantation System (OATS) procedure. The graft was harvested from the femoral condyle, implanted, and distracted with an external fixator. A follow-up MRI at 15 months postoperative demonstrated excellent graft incorporation. Similarly, Tsuda and colleagues[35] performed osteochondral autograft transplantation on 3 adolescent athletes, harvesting the graft from the lateral femoral trochlea. One patient with stage III and 2 patients with stage IV were selected. Computed tomography and MRI images were obtained postoperatively at 1 month and 24 months, which revealed incorporation of the graft.

Although no one method of surgical intervention has been agreed on, the practitioner is provided multiple treatment options. Many surgical methods have been described in the literature, ranging from joint debridement and arthoplasty to metatarsal head resection. All interventions have their strengths and weaknesses, ranging from pain relief and increased function to the complications of transfer metatarsalgia. However, the timing of treatment and the diagnosis of the stage of deformity are imperative to the overall success. Although uncommon, most practitioners will be faced with this diagnosis and treatment at some point during practice.

SUMMARY

Predislocation and Freiberg disease are 2 common pathologies that encapsulate most second MTPJ symptomatology. For foot and ankle clinicians, successful treatment of these syndromes has been less than favorable. A stout clinical examination and high degree of suspicion will often identify these debilitating syndromes in the early stages, where treatment options are more favorable. However, considering the chronic nature of second MTPJ pathology, presentation of these syndromes is often seen in advanced stages. Recent surgical techniques for predislocation syndrome and an array of surgical options for Freiberg disease have been developed with good promise, but further research is needed in this pathology.

REFERENCES

1. Deland JT, Lee KT, Sobel M, et al. Anatomy of the plantar plate and its attachments in the lesser metatarsal phalangeal joint. Foot Ankle Int 1995;16:480–6.
2. Medicino RW, Statler TK, Saltrick KR, et al. Predislocation syndrome: a review and retrospective analysis of eight patients. J Foot Ankle Surg 2001;40(1):214–24.
3. Coughlin MJ. Subluxation and dislocation of the second metatarsophalangeal joint. Orthop Clin North Am 1989;20:535–51.
4. Bhatia D, Myerson MS, Curtis MJ, et al. Anatomical restraints to dislocation of the second metatarsalphalangeal joint and assessment of a repair technique. J Bone Joint Surg Am 1994;76(9):1371–5.
5. Deland JT, Sung IH. The medial crossover toe: a cadaveric dissection. Foot Ankle Int 2000;21(5):375–8.

6. Ford LA, Collins KB, Christensen JC. Stabilization of the subluxed second meta-tarsalphalangeal joint: flexor tendon transfer verses primary repair of the plantar plate. J Foot Ankle Surg 1998;37(3):217–22.

7. Johnston RB, Smith J, Daniels T. The plantar plate of the lesser toes: an anatomical study of human cadavers. Foot Ankle Int 1994;15(5):276–82.

8. Cooper MT, Coughlin MJ. Sequential dissection for exposure of the second metatarsalphalangeal joint. Foot Ankle Int 2011;32(3):294–9.

9. Yu GV, Judge MS, Hudson JR, et al. Predislocation syndrome: progressive subluxation/dislocation of the lesser metatarsophalangeal joint. J Am Podiatr Med Assoc 2002;92(2):182–99.

10. Yu G, Judge M. Predislocation syndrome of the lesser metatarsophalangeal joint: a distinct clinical entity. Chapter 20. In: Camasta C, Vickers NS, Carter S, editors. Reconstructive surgery of the foot and leg, update 1995, vol. 99. Tucker (GA): The podiatry Institute Inc; 1995. p. 109–13.

11. Sferra J, Arndt S. The crossover toe and valgus toe deformity. Foot Ankle Clin 2011;16:609–20.

12. Kaz MD, Coughlin MJ. Crossover second toe: demographics, etiology, and radiographic assessment. Foot Ankle Int 2007;28(12):1223–37.

13. Coughlin MJ. Crossover second toe deformity. Foot Ankle 1987;8:29–39.

14. Coughlin MJ. When to suspect crossover second toe deformity. J Musculoskel Med 1987;4:39–48.

15. Coughlin MJ. Second metatarsophalangeal joint instability in the athlete. Foot Ankle 1993;14:309–19.

16. Panchbhavi V, Trevino S. Clinical tip: a new clinical sign associated with metatarsophalangeal joint synovitis of the lesser toes. Foot Ankle Int 2007;28:640–1.

17. Gazdag A, Cracchiolo A. A surgical treatment of patients with painful instability of the second metatarsophalangeal joint. Foot Ankle Int 1998;19:137–43.

18. Thompson FM, Deland JT. Flexor tendon transfer for metatarsophalangeal instability of the second toe. Foot Ankle 1993;14:385–8.

19. Reis ND, Karkabi S, Zinman C. Metatarsophalangeal joint dislocation after local steroid injection. J Bone Joint Surg Br 1989;71:864.

20. Noyes FR, Nussbaum NS, DeLucas JL, et al. Biomechanical and ultrastructure changes in ligaments and tendons after corticosteroid injection. J Bone Joint Surg Am 1975;57:876.

21. Haddad SL, Sabbagh RC, Resch S, et al. Results of flexor-extensor and extensor brevis tendon transfer for correction of crossover second toe deformity. Foot Ankle Int 1999;20:781–8.

22. Barca F, Acciaro AL. Surgical correction of crossover deformity of the second toe; a technique and tenodesis. Foot Ankle Int 2004;25:620–4.

23. Powless SH, Elze ME. Metatarsophalangeal joint capsule tears: an analysis by arthrography, a new classification system and surgical management. J Foot Ankle Surg 2001;40(6):116–21.

24. Weil L Jr, Sung W, Weil LS Sr, et al. Anatomic plantar plate repair using the Weil metatarsal osteotomy approach. Foot Ankle Spec 2011;4(3):145–50.

25. Coughlin MJ, Baumfeld DS, Nery C. Second MTP joint instability: grading of the deformity and description of surgical repair of capsular insufficiency. Phys Sportsmed 2011;39(3):132–41.

26. Gregg J, Silberstein M, Clark C, et al. Plantar plate repair and Weil osteotomy for metatarsophalangeal joint instability. Foot Ankle Surg 2007;13(3):116–21.

27. Freiberg AH. Infraction of the second metatarsal bone, a typical injury. Surg Gynecol Obstet 1914;19:191.

28. Cerrato RA. Freiberg's disease. Foot Ankle Clin 2011;16:647.
29. Ashman CJ, Rosemary KJ, Yu JS. Forefoot pain involving the metatarsal region: differential diagnosis with MR imaging. Radiographics 2001;21:1427.
30. Smillie IS. Treatment of Freiberg's infraction. Proc R Soc Med 1967;60:29–31.
31. El-Tayeby HM. Freiberg's infraction: a new surgical procedure. J Foot Ankle Surg 1998;37:23–4.
32. Gauthier G, Elbaz R. Freiberg's infraction: a subchondral bone fatigue fracture. A new surgical treatment. Clin Orthop Relat Res 1979;(142):93–5.
33. Edmonson MC, Sherry KR, Afolyan J, et al. Case series of 17 modified Weil's osteotomies for Freiberg's and Kohler's II AVN, with AOFAS scoring pre and post-operatively. Foot Ankle Surgery 2011;17:19–24.
34. DeVries GJ, Amoit RA, Cummings P, et al. Freiberg's infraction of the second metatarsal treated with autologous osteochondral transplantation and external fixation. J Foot Ankle Surg 2008;47:565–9.
35. Tsuda E, Ishibashi Y, Yamamoto Y, et al. Osteochondral autograft transplantation for advanced stage Freiberg disease in adolescent athletes. Am J Sports Med 2011;39:2470–5.

First Metatarsophalangeal Joint Arthrodesis; What is the Best Fixation Option?

A Critical Review of the Literature

Joseph R. Treadwell, DPM

KEYWORDS

- First metatarsophalangeal joint • Arthrodesis • Fusion

KEY POINTS

- First metatarsophalangeal joint arthrodesis can be accomplished using many forms of fixation.
- A review of the literature provides a starting point for what needs to be assessed and what questions need to be asked.
- In vivo and in vitro studies attempt to provide answers but frequently reveal shortcomings in the evidence to date.

It seems easy to identify the best fixation method for arthrodesis of the first metatarsophalangeal joint (MTPJ). Take the strongest fixation that can be easily applied that provides the highest union rate, at the cheapest cost, with the fewest associated complications, and that allows the patient the greatest degree of freedom. However, even with an abundance of literature available, this choice may not be clear.

In this article, the question of the best fixation technique for first MTPJ arthrodesis is not related to revisional surgery, osteopenic osseous segments, patients with distinctive comorbidities, or complex reconstructions.

The goals of first MTPJ fusion include improving function of the patient or decreasing disability and reducing pain. Fixation can be evaluated by its ability to help achieve these goals with the following tenets:

- Achieving high fusion rate
- Lack of unique fixation-specific complications
- Ease of application
- Cost-effectiveness
- Maintain apposition and position of bone segments

Private practice, Foot and Ankle Specialists of CT, 6 Germantown Road, Danbury, CT 06810, USA
E-mail address: jtread6692@aol.com

Clin Podiatr Med Surg 30 (2013) 327–349
http://dx.doi.org/10.1016/j.cpm.2013.04.008
0891-8422/13/$ – see front matter © 2013 Elsevier Inc. All rights reserved.

- Does not require ancillary procedure for removal
- Allows reproducible results
- Allows early limb dependency with ankle mobilization (heel weight bearing)

The literature shows that obtaining a high fusion rate, more than 90%, does not depend on 1 type of fixation.[1–19,21,22] **Table 1** shows in vivo fusion rates associated with various forms of fixation.[1–19,21,22] Articles were selected from studies in the post-2000 literature with more than 15 attempted arthrodeses. Dissection techniques, joint surface preparation, postoperative protocols, and postoperative foot protection varied among studies. Sample sizes reflected in the chart are not necessarily what the study abstracts listed. Only those fusions included in the final analyses were considered. Nonunion rates charted were calculated on failed fusions divided by total attempted fusions. Some studies used patient numbers instead of joints fused, which could be problematic in bilateral cases if both feet failed to fuse. Patient-based calculations of bilateral nonunions can provide an inaccurate nonunion rate for total attempted fusions. Some studies compared multiple fixation techniques; however, those cohorts with small sample sizes (eg, 1–6) were excluded from the chart.

Terminology has different meanings between studies. Crossed screws can indicate bicortical purchase or intramedullary screw tip position.[7] In the same way, one screw technique could indicate bicortical lag screw or intramedullary screw technique. Single-screw technique includes proximal to distal orientation and vice versa, as well as intramedullary and bicortical purchase.[1,7,9,14] The text of articles does not always identify screw orientation or cortical purchase and images are sometimes the only identifier. Screw sizes among reviewed studies ranged from 2.1 mm to 6.5 mm, solid and cannulated screws. There are no in vitro studies that compare traditional crossed-screw fixation in cannulated versus solid or crossed-screw fixation versus 2 parallel screws from any orientation. There are also no current studies that compared crossed screws of different diameters. In vitro studies may help determine optimal screw sizes for the most stable construct, because surgeons have used screws as small as 2.7 mm cannulated.[23] Few in vivo studies compare fixation constructs tested within in vitro studies.

In some studies comparing different fixation techniques, postoperative protocols and protective footwear varied between groups, which could have altered outcomes and makes nonunion rate comparisons less valid.[9,19] Within studies testing one type of fixation, orientation of the device varied from patient to patient, as shown in radiographic examples that can affect the strength of fixation and validity and reliability of the study.[11] Some studies totaled up to 14 surgeons, which also affects the variability and reliability of the study.[7]

Spherical reamers were referred to in various studies as conical, dome-shaped, convex and concave, and ball and cup.[8,12,13]

Studies comparing locked versus nonlocked plates commonly used plates of different designs, widths, thicknesses, and materials, with different screw orientation and different screw sizes within the same study preventing a clear distinction between the two technologies.[19,22] Although some studies found locking plate design superior, others did not.

There has yet to be a determination of whether plates with H-shaped design, in-line screw holes, or a variation of the two are best in the first MTPJ. Some studies fail to identify, via text or imaging, the fixation used or screw sizes, precluding comparison with other studies.[3]

More concerning is the interpretation of fusion when the imaging provided shows a lack of healing, which calls into question whether the specified fusion rate is accurate.[14] Other studies indicate they are testing one type of construct but their imaging shows another.[5,14]

Even the most basic of fixation studies related to K-wire and Steinman fixation fail to definitively establish long-term sequelae of crossing the interphalangeal joint (IPJ) for fusion of the first MTPJ. If IPJ arthritis does not develop after removal of percutaneous fixation, these techniques become a feasible option because they can be buried to eliminate the transcutaneous pathway for infection and removed via a stab incision at a later time when they do cross the IPJ. This ancillary procedure prevents this technique from meeting the parameters mentioned previously but can still provide a desired outcome.

Terminology in published reports, such as locking or crossed screws, or used in reviewing nonunion rates, provides little information when comparing efficacy of fixation constructs at obtaining an appropriate outcome. **Table 1** shows a comparison between studies; however, at times it is the sum of the articles that provides the desired information and not just the individual study.

The review of the following studies is not necessarily to compare studies but to acknowledge tenets that better assist the surgeon to assess first MTPJ arthrodesis techniques. An author cannot always capture the breadth of a referenced study because it would be too tenuous and could distract from the goals and objectives of their article. Readers need to critically review the literature on their own.

IN VIVO STUDIES

A retrospective study by Bennett and Sabetta,[13] 2009, incorporated more consistency among variables than most in vivo studies. A single surgeon performed 233 cases using 1 joint preparation technique, manual contouring, with an identical postoperative protocol for all patients. A toe spica was applied and patients were non–weight bearing for 1 week. At 1 week, patients were placed into an Aircast SP walker boot and allowed to weight bear on the heel for 6 weeks. The walker was weaned away as the patients' pain allowed. No bilateral procedures were done. One plate system, Accutrak first MTPJ fusion system, was used identified as nonlocking. Screws 3.5 mm cortical and 4.0 mm cancellous were used, although it was not identified whether the same screw type was inserted into the same hole position on each plate. Their union rate was 98.7%. This study has enough standardization among variables in tandem with a large sample population to allow the reader to draw some basic conclusions related to the combination of joint surface preparation, fixation construct, and postoperative protocol used. Because these variables differ within studies with low sample populations, it is difficult to assert reliability and validity. Bilateral procedures can affect weight bearing and load strain differently than unilateral procedures affecting outcome. Most studies include bilateral cases.

A prospective study by Choudhary and colleagues,[4] 2004, used 2 memory compression staples positioned at 90° to each other with the joint surfaces manually contoured. All surgeries were performed by 1 surgeon. The union rate was 96.7%. The joint preparation technique, fixation, and postoperative protocol were the same for all patients. Patients were allowed to fully weight bear in a rigid-soled shoe from surgical day 1. The investigators included their fenestration technique using a 2-mm drill. Although this fenestration technique has the potential to incorporate autogenous graft between the surfaces interface, its impact on fusion rate has not been determined at this site. Although the study tried to limit variability, the reader can appreciate additional variables that could affect fusion rates among studies. They did not define full weight bearing, so the reader is left to assume they meant that the patient had no restrictions on loading the forefoot.

Table 1
In vivo studies

Author/Year/ Country	Fixation	Nonunion Rate (%)	Sample Population (N)	Joint Preparation Technique	Postoperative WB Status	Protective Footwear	Average Range of Time to Fusion (wk)	Average Range of Follow-up (mo)
Agoropoulos et al,[1] 2001/GR	3.5 cortical screw	3	62	Cone-shaped CR	NWB 2 wk HWB day 15	Aluminum padded splint	9–12	258 (24–372)
Santini & Walker,[2] 2001/ United Kingdom	LS + Luhr Vitallium mandibular plate 2.7/2.1 BCS	3	33	Spherical CR	DNR	Wooden shoe	7.59 (5–20)	25.4 (12–39)
Sharma & Geary,[3] 2002/United Kingdom	CS SNR	10	30	Planar	FWB after day 2	Splint 2 d. Plaster slipper cast after 2 d	DNR	77 (4–104)
Choudhary et al,[4] 2004/United Kingdom	2 staples	3	30	MJSM	FWB	Rigid-soled shoe	8	25 (11–35)
Aslam & Ribbans,[5] 2005/United Kingdom	LS + Luhr Vitallium mandibular plate	3	33	Spherical CR	NWB 2 wk. HWB 4 wk. FWB as tolerated	Special shoe	DNR	28 (16–45)
Brodsky et al,[6] 2005/United States	Parallel 3.5 bicortical cortical screws	0	60	MJSM	NWB 4 wk. Wear shoe while sleeping	Surgical shoe	DNR	44 (12–102)
Patil et al,[7] 2005/ United Kingdom	CS	0	28	MJSM	HWB or NWB. WB as tolerated n = 6	Plaster cast. Thermoplastic splint.	DNR	DNR
Goucher & Coughlin,[8] 2006/United States	IS + dorsal plate 2.7/3.0 screws	8	53	CR	HWB and lateral foot	Toe spica wrap and Surgical shoe	12	16 (12–24)

Study	Technique	n (SS=0/SS+P=6)	n (SS=16/SS+P=18)	Type	Weightbearing	Immobilization	Time to fusion	Follow-up
Sharma et al,[9] 2007/United Kingdom	SS vs SS with dorsal plate 2.7/2.1 bicortical	SS = 0 SS + P = 6	SS = 16 SS + P = 18	Planar	HWB	SS Plaster bootie, SS + P surgical shoe	SS 12 (8-16) SS + P 11 (9-18)	34.8 (21.6-48)
Grondal & Stark,[10] 2008/SW	CS	5	22	Cup and cone	WB as tolerated	Slipper cast	DNR	DNR
Mah & Banks,[11] 2009/United States	Crossed K-wires	9	22	MJSM	FWB	Padded surgical shoe	Average 9-12	DNR
Bennett & Sabetta,[13] 2009/United States	First MTPJ fusion NL plate 3.5 cortical/4.0 cancellous	1	233	MJSM	NWB week 1 Heel WB 6 wk	Walker boot	DNR	12 mo minimum all patients
Wassink & van den Oever,[14] 2009/NL	Single IM LS	4	109	Planar	NWB 3 d Crutch assisted heel WB 2 wk FWB week 3	Cast day 3-2 wk BK cast/stiff-soled shoe week 3	104 fused within 8 wk	59 (7-114)
Kumar et al,[15] 2010/United Kingdom	LS + dorsal MTP NL plate	2	46	CR	FWB	Surgical shoe	Average.3.1 mo	23 (14-37)
Bauer et al,[16] 2010/FR	3.0 cancellous CS	3	32	Percutaneous	FWB	Surgical shoe	(6-24)	12 mo minimum all patients
Besse et al,[17] 2010/FR	3 staples	6	54	CR	HWB	Slipper cast	Average 8	38.6 (22-56)
Sung et al,[18] 2010/United States	Dorsal LP + LS	6	47	CR	NWB 2 wk WB as tolerated after week 2	Splint 2 wk Protective boot after week 2	7.9 (6-10)	17.7 (3-68)
Hunt et al,[19] 2011/United States	Titanium LP + LS Steel NL + LS 2.7/3.2 screws	LP 23 NL 11	LP 73 NL 107	CR	HWB 2 wk + WB as tolerated HWB 6 wk most	Walking boot or surgical shoe	DNR	6 mo minimum

(continued on next page)

Table 1
(continued)

Author/Year/Country	Fixation	Nonunion Rate (%)	Sample Population (N)	Joint Preparation Technique	Postoperative WB Status	Protective Footwear	Average Range of Time to Fusion (wk)	Average Range of Follow-up (mo)
Roukis et al,[20] 2012/United States	Flexible titanium IM nails + staple	3	195 women	Planar	HWB and lateral foot	Surgical shoe	DNR	10 (6.5–13.5)
Hyer et al,[21] 2012/United States	NL NL + LS LP LP + LS	NL 5 NL + LS 14 LP 8 LP + LS 4	NL 43 NL + L 14 LP 36 LP + LS 45	CR	NWB 1 wk WB week 2–7	Splint week 1 Walking boot weeks 2–7	NL 8.4 NL + LS 8 LP 9.6 LP + LS 9 Averages	NL 12.25 NL + LS 12.2 LP 9.82 LP + LS 4.59 Averages
Dening & van Erve,[22] 2012/NL	LS 2.7 CS 2.7 N NLP + LS 2.7	LS 29 CS 10 NLP 0 NL + LS 7	LS 24 CS 21 NL 13 NL + LS 14	Planar	HWB	Forefoot-relieving surgical shoe	DNR	All patients Minimum 3 mo

Abbreviations: BCS, bicortical screw; BK, below knee; CR, conical reamer; CS, crossed screws; DNR, did not report; FR, France; FWB, Full weight bearing; GR, Greece; HWB, heel weight bearing; IM, intramedullary; IS, interfragmentary screw; LP, locking plate; LS, lag screw; MJSM, manual joint surface maintained; NL, nonlocking plate; NL under country, Netherlands; NWB, non–weight bearing; P, plate; SNR, size not reported; SS, single screw; WB, weight bearing.

Brodsky and colleagues,[6] 2005, incorporated a functional assessment as well as a functional questionnaire measuring activities of daily living. Their study incorporated the same joint surface preparation, fixation technique, and postoperative protocol for all patients. Their union rate was 100% for parallel screw fixation directed from the dorsal first metatarsal to the plantar aspect of the proximal phalanx with the joint surfaces manually contoured. Imaging for their surgical site showed the least amount of soft tissue dissection while allowing full exposure of the joint surfaces compared with all open techniques listed in the bibliography that provided joint exposure images. Technique images from other studies included spherical reaming systems, crossed and single screws, plates, and staples. Patients were in postoperative shoes for 7 to 8 weeks. Weight bearing was prohibited for the first 4 weeks with walker or crutch assistance. The addition of the functional assessment and questionnaire provide additional assessments that could be considered when assessing the best fixation. Patient satisfaction surveys provide end data information, but functional assessments and information may reveal differences among techniques, related to both fixation and dissection, that could affect long-term outcomes. Brodsky and colleagues'[6] study suggested directing the patient to wear the shoe even while sleeping. Few, if any, studies identify some form of surgical site protection while sleeping. Pressure from sheets, stomach sleeping, and active sleepers have the potential to apply load to the fixation, which could lead to failure.

Wassink and van den Oever,[14] 2009, reviewed 109 fusions fixated with a single 3.5 intramedullary cortical screw with planar joint resection directed from the medial metatarsal laterally into the phalangeal medullary canal. Although they had a 96% fusion rate, 78% (85 feet) required removal of the screw because of irritation. On reviewing their technique, there was no comment of countersinking and it appeared on imaging that screws were inserted without the head fully contacting the cortex. Patients were placed in a cast after 3 days and walked with crutches, just touching the heel to the ground. Patients were allowed to fully weight bear on a below-knee walking cast or surgical shoe after 2 weeks. Of concern is that the investigators present an image that is supposed to show union of the fusion site but is more consistent with a nonhealed site, raising concern for the reliability of their fusion assessment.

Not all studies related to fixation constructs are designed to show the best fusion rate. Even when different fixation constructs with different postoperative protocols and foot protection are used within the same study, important inferences can be obtained. Sharma and colleagues,[9] 2007, in an in vivo study, evaluated fusion rate differences between a single compression screw (100%) and a compression screw with dorsal plate (94%) with planar joint resection for both constructs. The single-screw group wore plaster booties with heel weight bearing, whereas the plate-and-screw group was placed in surgical shoes. Patient demographics and sample sizes were similar in both groups. There were 2 surgeons, and fusion position ranges were identified as well as complications. Although not all variables were able to be analyzed and the sample sizes were small (screws n = 16, plates n = 18), they provided enough data to show no significant difference in time to clinical and radiographic fusion by adding a dorsal plate to a single compression screw as described.

A prospective study by Goucher and Coughlin,[8] 2006, included other variables that should be considered when assessing fixation constructs. They reviewed 54 fusions using dome-shaped reamers with the same fixation construct and postoperative protocol for all patients. They included the Visual Analog Scale (VAS), American Orthopaedic Foot and Ankle Society (AOFAS) scoring assessments, preoperative and postoperative interphalangeal joint (IPJ) and metatarsocuneiform joint arthritis scores, subjective pain ratings, ambulatory capacity, and preoperative and postoperative first ray angles. Although IPJ arthritis is commonly stated in other articles to be of no significance, this assumption has yet to be determined by long-term studies. Goucher and Coughlin[8] maintained patients in a postoperative shoe for 12 weeks. Although their fusion rate was 92%, their time to fusion averaged 12 weeks, which is longer than many other studies with differing fixation constructs (see **Table 1**), and their follow-up was limited to 1 year. More important than their time to fusion or fusion rate are the additional parameters they assessed. The best fixation is not necessarily the one that simply produces the highest fusion rate. The fixation construct should also show an overall superiority in many of the variables/assessments and long-term outcomes reviewed in this study, which is exemplified by the inability of a specific fixation construct to maintain the ideal fusion position or it causing symptomatic IPJ arthritis.

Agoropoulos and colleagues,[1] 2001, performed a study using a single 3.5-mm cortical screw with a cone-shaped joint surface configuration. The screw was oriented from the medial proximal phalanx into the lateral metatarsal. Patients were non–weight bearing for 2 weeks and protected by a malleable aluminum splint followed by full heel weight bearing until radiologic union was noted. Unprotected weight bearing was typically allowed 3 months later. Although they had a 96% union rate, their study was of interest because of its longitudinal nature. Follow-up ranged from 2 to 31 years with an average of 25 years, which allowed assessment of long-term sequelae as a result of fusion, such as IPJ arthritis and pseudarthrosis tolerance. The patient who developed bilateral pseudarthrosis had not developed pain in either foot 10 years after surgery. Although other studies also comment on asymptomatic nonunions in the short term, the study by Agoropoulos and colleagues[1] shows how that pain-free status may continue over time. They also noted that, although IPJ arthritis is a common radiologic finding, it did not produce subjective complaints. The development of IPJ arthritis may not be a significant variable in evaluating fixation techniques because it may be related to the procedure itself.

Hyer and colleagues,[21] in 2012, reviewed 4 fixation constructs in 138 fusions: static plate, static plate with lag screw, locked plate, and locked plate with lag screw. Their joint preparation, conical reamers, and postoperative course (non–weight bearing week 1 in a splint followed by a high-tide walking boot for 6 additional weeks) were similar for all patients. They commented that "a standard titanium 4-hole MTP plate" was used in all patients, but provided imaging that showed additional 6-hole plates used, with some imaging showing all 6 holes filled. Three different plate designs were shown with different screw positions and orientations with 2 different types of headless screws used as the lag screw. They commented that no biologics were used to augment fusion, but a 2-mm drill was used to fenestrate the fusion surfaces. This type of fenestration has the potential to pull autogenous bone into the fusion site. Although their fusion rates were 86% to 96% for the different constructs, no comparison can be made related to locking versus nonlocking technology with or without lag screw supplementation as a result of these disparities in plate and screw design.

Hunt and colleagues[19] in 2011 performed a study comparing locked (n = 73) versus nonlocked technology (n = 107). Their union rate for locked technology was 93% and, for nonlocking technology, 95%. Their joint surface preparation (domed reamer) was the same for all patients; however, their postoperative protocol was not consistent for all patients. Two different plate constructs of different materials were used. Different plate screw-hole orientation and position, as well as different screw sizes, were used. Different types of lag screws were also shown on imaging. Within their operative technique was their dissection description, which included complete release of the soft tissues about the metatarsal head to allow for reaming. This description acknowledges the significant dissection associated with conical reamers and correlates with images supplied by other studies. Their union rates were still significantly high, which may indicate that periosteal capsular stripping may not have a profound impact on union rate.

Patil and colleagues[7] performed a study with the conclusion that: "Fusion rates are higher when two screws are used for fixation rather than one. Staples and K-wire fixation have a higher rate of non-union. Non-unions are often symptomatic." Their sample populations with a total of 56 feet included 2 screws in 31 feet (28 crossed and 3 parallel), 1 screw in 18 feet, staples in 6 feet, and K-wires in 1 foot. Their union rates were 100% for 2 screws, 77.8% for 1 screw, and 0% for staples and K-wires. They incorporated 2 different joint surface preparation techniques. Three different weight-bearing protocols were used: heel weight bearing, non–weight bearing, and weight bearing as tolerated. Two different foot protection devices were used. Imaging of crossed screws had the appearance of 1 bicortical and 1 intramedullary screw, whereas imaging of the single-screw technique was an intramedullary lag screw directed from the medial proximal phalanx into the first metatarsal shaft. There was no operative technique description or imaging of K-wire or staple fixation. Fourteen surgeons were involved in the study. They comment in discussion that "results quite clearly demonstrate that using staples or a single screw for fixation had a higher failure rate irrespective of the surgeon performing the operation." Although this statement is accurate for their study, their results are not consistent with other studies regarding single-screw, staple, and K-wire fixation, and their conclusion does not apply beyond their study.[1,5,10,12]

A review of a few articles shows the difficulty in a comparison of union rates associated with differing fixation constructs. Studies provide a good-faith estimate of the fusion rate and outcome with the specific fixation construct and protocol incorporated by the author. The longitudinal nature of a study allows a better evaluation for complications such as removal because of irritation. Assessments may provide a better appreciation for the perioperative experience of the patient.

IN VITRO STUDIES

In vitro studies provide the best opportunity to compare strength of fixation as well as whether specific surface preparation techniques enhance stability of the fusion site. Failure of fixation can result from a single force that exceeds the strength of the fixation construct, resulting in sudden failure, or repetitive forces of smaller magnitude that result in failure via a fatigue process.[24] Nonunions typically present without any significant osseous or fixation shift occurring more likely from the latter failure mode. As more surgeons allow patients the ability to weight bear after surgery, without any means of offloading the first MTPJ, repetitive forces can be applied across the fusion site.

Table 2 identifies the most commonly referenced in vitro studies for fixation of first MTPJ fusions.[23,25–31] Even among these studies there was not a consensus for the best surface preparation technique to enhance fixation stiffness and strength to failure.[23,25–31] Most studies focused on testing various fixation constructs with 1 joint preparation technique, which allows a better comparison of fixation constructs, but does not allow comparison of joint resection techniques. Conical reaming, cup and cone, manual debridement maintaining joint shape, and planar resection were used for surface preparation throughout the studies cited.

Bone segments among in vitro studies vary in that some use synthetic material and others use cadaver bone, with varying testing apparatus making failure force comparison between studies less optimal. The manner in which constructs were stabilized and loaded for testing varied between studies.

Table 2
In vitro studies

Author/Year/Country	Fixation	Surface Preparation	Joint Set Position Dorsiflexion/Valgus Degrees	Load Distance to Joint (mm)	Load to Failure (Mean, Newtons)
Sykes & Hughes,[25] 1986, United Kingdom	4-mm AO screw	Dome and socket	20/20	NG	12.9
	4-mm AO screw	Planar	20/20	NG	23.7
Curtis et al,[23] 1991, United States	Crossed K-wires	Planar	25/15	25	40.2
	1/4 tubular 5-hole to 6-hole plate, 3.5 cortical screws	Planar	25/15	25	20.6
	3.5-mm bicortical screw from metatarsal-phalanx	Planar	25/15	25	12.6
	3.5-mm bicortical screw from metatarsal-phalanx	Cone shaped	25/15	25	91.2
Rongstad,[26] 1994, United States	AO 4-mm bicortical cancellous screw (phalanx to metatarsal) + K-wire	Planar	25/15	21	97/147
	4.5-mm Herbert bone screw (90° to joint) + K-wire	Planar	25/15	21	154
	Miniplate (2.7-mm bicortical screws) + K-wire	Planar	25/15	21	242
	Steinman pin + K-wire	Planar	25/15	21	131
Buranosky et al,[27] 2001, United States	Vitallium 6-hole plate (2.7 screws, 3 on each side) + 2.7-mm lag screw	SR	20/15	12	180
	Crossed 2.7-mm bicortical screws	SR	20/15	12	130

Study	Fixation				
Neufeld et al,[28] 2002, United States	2 memory compression staples + K-wire	Planar	25/15	End of phalanx	~35
	Dorsal plate (3.5 bicortical screws) + K-wire	Planar	25/15	End of phalanx	63
	4-mm cancellous crossed bicortical screws	Planar	25/15	End of phalanx	79
Molloy et al,[29] 2003, United States	Crossed 4-mm partially threaded cannulated cancellous screws	MJP	25–30/10–15	End of phalanx	100
	6.5 partially threaded cancellous IM screw + K-wire	MJP	25–30/10–15	End of phalanx	149
Politi et al,[30] 2003, United States	3.5-mm bicortical screw, phalanx to metatarsal	SR	20/10	PC	1870 N-Mm moment
	Crossed 0.062" K-wires	SR	20/10	PC	304 N-Mm moment
	Vitallium miniplate 3.5 screws + 3.5 cortical lag screw	SR	20/10	PC	4958 N-Mm moment
	Miniplate 3.5 cortical screws	SR	20/10	PC	397 N-Mm moment
	3.5-mm bicortical screw, phalanx to metatarsal	Planar	20/10	PC	3030 N-Mm moment
Faraj et al,[31] 2007, United Kingdom	Circumferential wire	Synthetic rods	NG	20	60
	Screw fixation (not described)	Synthetic rods	NG	20	413

Abbreviations: MJP, manual joint preparation; NG, not given; PC, center of phalangeal condyles; SR, spherical reaming system.

Sykes and Hughes,[25] 1986, did a study with 15 pairs of cadavers. A template was used to position all specimens in 20° of dorsiflexion and 20° of valgus. The failure point was the point at which the fixation construct could no longer maintain the applied load to the proximal phalanx. They compared AO 4-mm screw (with both planar cuts and dome-and-socket surface preparation) with an external fixation device and 2 wire configurations associated with planar joint resection. Screw orientation was directed from the proximal phalanx into the metatarsal with the tip resting on the cortex but not penetrating it (intramedullary). Planar cuts provided a stronger load to failure (23.7 N/mm) versus dome and socket (12.9 N/mm). The investigators stated that the dome-and-socket joint surface behaved as a ball-and-socket joint, allowing the proximal phalanx to roll dorsally away from the metatarsal where the planar cuts failed when the fixation devices cut out. They also reviewed an external fixation construct (5 N/mm) and 2 wire suture configurations (2.3 N/mm and 2.2 N/mm). The weakest part of the compression screw fixation was at the bony flange of the proximal phalanx. Eleven of the compression screw specimens failed by the screw head region snapping through the flange of the phalanx, with the other 4 failures occurring by the threads pulling out of the metatarsal bone. The screws were tightened manually by the same surgeon who compressed until he thought that they were equally tight, as opposed to using instrumentation to measure compression force during application. They did not supply details of the rate load that was applied or from what distance from the MTPJ it was applied.

An in vitro study by Curtis and colleagues,[23] 1991, is commonly cited to show that power conical reaming (PCR) systems are superior to planar resection at increasing stability to the joint fixation construct. They tested 10 fresh pairs of cadaver specimens. The conical reaming technique from this study is not similar to the cup-and-cone/domed/ball-and-cup/spherical systems used today. The system from the Curtis and colleagues[23] study fashioned a significantly long metatarsal cone that penetrated into a deeply reamed phalangeal component. Reaming systems commonly used at present are more spherical in nature. In this study they tested crossed K-wire fixation, dorsal plate system (DPS), and bicortical 3.5-mm interfragmentary cortical screw (IFS) with planar resection against power conically reamed surfaces fixated with 3.5-mm bicortical screws. The PCR construct (mean 91.2 N/mm) with single lag screw was significantly more stable than the dorsal plate (mean, 20.6 N/mm) and single lag screw (mean, 28.2 N/mm) with planar cuts. The PCR and K-wire with planar resection showed no difference in initial stability. The PCR group (22.0 N/mm) had a higher mean load than the K-wires (16.3 N/mm) to produce 1-mm and 2-mm displacement and load to failure (mean 79.4 N/mm and 40.2 N/mm) respectively. The figures of 1 to 2 mm of displacement between the PCR and K-wire constructs were not statistically significant. The IFS (mean 28.2 N) with planar cuts was significantly stronger than DPS (20.6 N) at load to failure. The DPS failed with bending at the joint level. A 5-hole or 6-hole AO one-quarter tubular plate was used. The distal 2 screws were filled in the phalangeal side. The first proximal screw hole in the metatarsal side was left open and the next 2 holes were filled in the metatarsal for a 6-hole plate. The narrowest amount of plate segment was positioned directly over the joint line in a 6-hole plate because an open screw hole (fourth screw hole) was positioned here. A 5-hole plate would leave an unfilled hole directly over the joint line. Plate technology has shown that plate width contributes to stiffness against bending, which may explain why the IFS was more stable than the DPS in this study. Within this study they identified that load was applied plantar to dorsal 25 mm from the joint line at a rate of 2 mm/min until failure of fixation occurred. Failure was at 5 mm of displacement. The joints were fixed at 25° of dorsiflexion and 15° of valgus, measured with a goniometer. Although their conclusions were correct for the constructs they tested, the reaming system is not a common shape in modern systems and the plate and design position do not apply to first MTPJ plate systems currently used. This study does not support the premise that current spherical reaming systems create a joint surface that provides more stability than planar resection.

Rongstad and colleagues,[26] 1994, performed a study with 18 matched pairs of cadaveric specimens. They compared 4 fixation constructs, 4.0 AO bicortical cancellous screw from the medial phalanx to lateral metatarsal, 4.5 cannulated Herbert intramedullary screw perpendicular to the fusion site, 6-hole 41-mm dorsal miniplate with 2.7-mm bicortical screws, and 2.4-mm (3/32 inch) Steinman pin longitudinally placed down the phalanx and exiting the plantar metatarsal cortex, all stabilizing planar resected surfaces. Each fixation construct was supplemented with a 1.1-mm (0.045 inch) K-wire placed across the fusion site. The fusion sites were fixed at 25° of dorsiflexion and 15° of valgus. Load was applied 21 mm from the joint line directed dorsally from the plantar phalanx at a rate of 1 mm/min. The point at which the observed force began to decrease was defined as the failure point. The miniplate (mean 316 N) had a 2.5 times greater force to failure and 3.1 times (118 N/mm) greater initial stiffness than the 4.0 screw (mean 95 N and 30 N/mm), both differences being statistically significant. The Herbert screw (mean 207 N) was 2.3 times stronger in force to failure than the 4.0 screw, which was statistically significant. Although the Herbert screw also had a greater initial stiffness, this was not statistically significant. The Steinman pin and 4.0 screw had similar values. There are many points of concern for the study presented. The supplemental K-wire that was included for each fixation was not standardized in its placement with each construct. It also served to prevent rotation that could prevent an initial failure process within a construct. How this affected the final measurements cannot be predicted. The Herbert bone screw guidewire was inserted into the metatarsal from the joint site out the plantar metatarsal shaft, then retrograded through the medullary canal of the phalanx so that it was perpendicular to the arthrodesis surfaces. This application is not practical in a clinical setting and would prove significantly more challenging than other constructs with better strength studies. The Steinman pins were inserted from the phalanx exiting the plantar metatarsal cortex. In the clinical setting, this would mean crossing the IPJ. Although postsurgical changes of the IPJ have not proved to be of clinical significance in the subjective reporting of pain by the patient, this has been with fixation that did not violate the IPJ.

Buranosky and colleagues,[27] 2001, performed an in vitro study with 12 matched pair of cadaver specimens comparing crossed 2.7-mm screws versus 6-hole Vitallium alloy plate. The plate incorporated 2.7 screws, 3 screws in each segment, with a supplemental interfragmentary screw. The MTPJ was set at 20° of dorsiflexion and 15° of abduction with the load applied from the plantar aspect of the phalanx vertically 12 mm from the joint line at a rate of 2 mm/min. Load to failure was identified graphically at the point where linear progression of applied force peaked and then decreased. The plate construct (mean, 121 N/mm) was significantly stiffer than the crossed screws (mean, 72 N/mm) from 0 to 1 mm of displacement but not from 1 to 2 mm of displacement. The plate construct (mean, 180 N) was also statistically stiffer than the crossed screws (mean, 130 N) in load to failure. This study did not assess the 2 constructs under repetitive load conditions assessing for repetitive stress strength. Unlike the study by Curtis and colleagues,[23] the plate in this study had full-width solid material over the MTPJ. Their crossed screw technique had both screws inserted from distal to proximal. Their screws were 2.7 mm in diameter and how this corresponds with 3.5-mm and 4.0-mm screws cannot be determined. How this compares with crossed screws inserted with both heads on the medial surfaces is unknown.

Neufeld and colleagues,[28] 2002, performed an in vitro study on 21 matched pairs of specimens. They compared 2 crossed bicortical cannulated screws, dorsal 5-hole one-third tubular plate with 3.5-mm bicortical screws and 2 compression staples all with planar cuts. They included a 1.6-mm (0.062-inch) K-wire with each construct to prevent rotation. The wire was positioned in the same orientation with each construct. Toes were fixed in 25° of dorsiflexion and 15° of valgus. Load was applied at the distal end of the proximal phalanx. Load was applied at a rate of 2 mm/min. A 2-mm gap was defined as the point of failure. They supplied bar graphs but no specific data for their stiffness and loads to failure. The average initial stiffness of the constructs was about 60 N/mm for plates, 75 N/mm for screws, and 25 N/mm for the staples. The two cannulated screws were 3 times stiffer than the staples and although the screws were stiffer than the plate, the difference was not statistically significant. The crossed screws and plate constructs failed at significantly higher loads than the staples. The approximate range of failure for the constructs was about 70 N to 120 N for plates, 70 N to 105 N for screws and about 20 N to 45 N for staples. Concerns with this study include that the load was applied at the distal end of each phalanx. Length difference among phalanges can increase the lever arm and this was not accounted for in the study. The crossed screws were not inserted in a commonly applied manner as seen in most in vivo studies for this time period. One screw was inserted from the dorsal medial metatarsal angled 45°to the fusion site, with the second screw inserted from the plantar medial side of the metatarsal into the proximal phalanx medullary canal as an interference fit. Screws were tightened to the discretion of the surgeon. The plates have the same issue as the study by Curtis and colleagues,[23] in that an open plate hole was centered over the joint line, placing the weakest part of the plate over the area of bending stress. Although the K-wire was inserted in a standard fashion for all constructs, it has the opportunity to falsely increase load to failure if the K-wire has a stronger load to failure than the construct being tested. This possibility is most concerning when testing the staples. They comment in their conclusion that none of the constructs they tested were strong enough to withstand load applied across the first MTPJ and external immobilization was required to achieve fusion. This tenet can be applied to any fixation construct and, if ignored, could lead to failure.

Molloy and colleagues,[29] 2002, in what they called an ex vivo study, used 5 pairs of cadaver specimens to compare 4.0-mm cannulated crossed screws with a 6.5 cannulated intramedullary screw. They fixed the first MTPJ at 25° to 30° of dorsiflexion and 10° to 15° of valgus. Joint surface preparation was through use of a burr to create hemispherical convex and concave surfaces. Load was applied at 1 mm/min from a plantar to dorsal direction between the distal condyles of the proximal phalanx. Failure was defined at 5 mm displacement. Stiffness was defined as the slope of the force versus deformation curve between 10 and 60 N of load. The 6.5-mm intramedullary group was significantly stiffer than the 4.0 interfragmentary group (18.7 ± 10.1 vs 10.2 ± 6.1 N/mm, respectively, mean ± standard deviation [SD]). The intramedullary group was also 50% stronger than the interfragmentary group (149 ± 88.2 vs 100.2 ± 70.8 N/mm, respectively, mean ± SD), although this difference was not significantly significant. The crossed screws were bicortical and positioned from the medial first metatarsal to the lateral phalanx and from the medial phalanx to the lateral metatarsal. The 6.5-mm cannulated intramedullary screw was inserted from the plantar surface of the neck of the first metatarsal into the phalanx near perpendicular to the joint line. The intramedullary 6.5-mm cannulated screw was supplemented with a 1.6-mm K-wire, whereas the crossed screws were not. This supplementation affects construct response to load. Difficulty in this technique occurs if the proximal phalanx shaft is too small for the 6.5 mm screw. Although two 3.5-mm screws could be used for smaller phalanges, it can still prove difficult with insertion as described. They did not test cyclic loading of the constructs. The angle of insertion can prove challenging because of the plantar soft tissues. If symptomatic nonunion occurs necessitating removal of the screw, removal would also prove more difficult than with other constructs.

Politi and colleagues,[30] 2003, compared 5 different constructs in synthetic bone models consisting of 40 specimens. The modulus of elasticity for compressive strength, tensile strength, and shear strength was stated to be similar to that of human cancellous bone. Detailed strength and modulus parameters were available. The 5 tested constructs included 3.5-mm cortical interfragmentary screw, crossed 1.6-mm (0.062 inch) K-wires, 3.5-mm cortical lag screw, and 4-hole dorsal Vitallium miniplate secured with three 3.5-mm cortical screws and no lag screw. All constructs secured conically reamed joint surfaces. The fifth construct was a single oblique 3.5-mm interfragmentary cortical lag screw securing joint surfaces prepared by planar resection. A jig was developed to allow reproducible placement of the 3.5-mm screws in all cases. The screws were directed from the medial proximal phalanx into the lateral metatarsal. The toes were fixed in 20° of dorsiflexion and 10° of valgus with 0° of rotation. A power analysis was performed to determine that 8 specimens per test group were needed, assuming a 10% synthetic bone population variance and desiring to detect a 20% significant difference in micro motion stiffness between groups. The mean gauge of displacement (the average of 8 cycles of collected data per trial) was calculated at an opening displacement of 0.9 mm with loading. The results of strength of fixation were dorsal plate with lag screw (4958.5 N/mm), planar surface with single lag screw (3030.2 N/mm), conical surface with single lag screw (1870.2 N/mm), dorsal plate only (397.5 N/mm), and K-wires (304.5 N/mm). The dorsal plate with lag screw was about 10 times more stable than the conically reamed surface. The planar surfaces with lag screw (3030.2 N/mm) were significantly stronger than the conical surface with lag screw (1870.2 N/mm). Although the plate and screw construct was the most stable of all techniques, they did not test a planar surface with the same plate-and-lag-screw construct. From their data, the planar surface preparation produced a more stable construct than the conically reamed surface with the same fixation. Their plate construct may have been similar in strength to the K-wires as a result of the shape and manner applied. The plate had extremely narrow width between holes, being about one-third the width of the screw holes. There was only 1 screw inserted into the proximal phalanx with the plate and an open screw hole over the joint line. This study was the only one to use a moment arm to convert force to moment. The distance from the center of the condyles of the distal phalanx to the center of the joint space was the moment arm. The lever arm value varied slightly between specimens. The moment arm length multiplied by the load determined the moment applied to the specimen.

A study by Faraj and colleagues,[31] 2007, tested circumferential wire-to-screw fixation in 66 synthetic (nylon) extruded rods 25 mm in diameter. Load was applied 20 mm from the simulated joint interface. Their testing model put the superior surface of the joint in tension and the inferior surface in compression. Load was applied at 1 mm/min. The screw fixation was stronger and stiffer than the wire fixation and failure by permanent deformation occurred at loads 6 times greater in the screw construct. They did not identify whether it was 1 or 2 screws or how the screw was positioned. They did not identify how the wire was applied. Images on the testing jig did not make this any clearer. This article offered no comparatively useful data.

Müller and colleagues,[32] 1970, comment that applying the plate to the tension side of the bone is essential for stable fixation. This is referenced when the authors wished to show a weakness or disadvantage of plate fixation compared with another construct. This comment is true regarding strength of fixation, but dorsally applied first

MTP plates commonly show stiffness and resistance to failure that are greater than other constructs. Dorsal plates also show a high fusion rate in in vivo studies, making this comment of questionable clinical relevance in this application.

In vitro studies should test constructs that are current. Even among the studies reviewed, it can be seen how application and testing method protocols can affect outcomes.

JOINT SURFACE PREPARATION

Joint surface preparation varies among studies, as shown in **Table 1**, and includes planar resection, manual preparation maintaining joint shape, and various PCR systems. In vitro studies show differing strength and strain results with planar versus cup-and-cone resection techniques. Some literature implies that cup-and-cone resection is more stable, but planar resection has proved more stable in side-by-side comparisons with the reamer systems currently in use. Ground reactive forces through the first MTPJ after surgery are mainly in the sagittal plane. It could be argued with heel-off that a planar joint creates resistance at the dorsal surface as the metatarsal declinates, and that a conical surface offers the opportunity for the phalanx to more readily pivot around the metatarsal head.

Current in vivo studies show many surgeons preferring conical reaming techniques or maintaining joint shape rather than planar resection. In addition to joint surface preparation's potential impact on joint stability and increasing bone-to-bone contact, maintaining length and vascularity are of concern and can affect fusion rates. Singh and colleagues[33] showed no significant statistical difference between a specific conical reamer system and flat-cut surface preparation on 6 paired cadaver feet related to postresection first ray length changes. Although they acknowledged that the size of their cohort groups may not have allowed statistically significant differences to be shown, they did minimize measurement errors in their approach by incorporating first and second ray relationships. Length alterations can lead to plantar pressure changes affecting stress distribution, which could be a factor in fusion rates depending on postoperative weight-bearing protocols.[34]

The impact of how and whether to fenestrate joint surfaces has not been investigated and is not always identified in studies. There are no studies that compare union rates of fenestrated versus nonfenestrated joint preparation with the same fixation. Nor are there studies that compare K-wire fenestration versus drill fenestration with the same fixation technique. Drill fenestration has the ability to draw autogenous bone between the joint surfaces; however, the significance of this has not been assessed in first MTPJ arthrodesis.

JOINT POSITION AND STRAIN

Weight bearing without restriction can allow about 119% of body weight to pass through the first metatarsal head.[35] At toe-off the metatarsal head can incur a load of more than 50% (350 N) of body weight.[36] To allow unrestricted weight bearing after fusion, the fixation needs to withstand this load. Fixation must also be able to prevent joint motion from isometric contraction of the muscles about the first MTPJ. Actuation of muscles and tendons about the first MTPJ may prevent bone loss and assist in the healing process.[37] Isometric flexor hallucis longus (FHL) function provides forces that act across the great toe.[38] With complete immobilization of the limb, bone strength can diminish.

A robotic cadaver study by Bayomy and colleagues[39] studied the fused dorsiflexion angle and its impact on pressures under the first metatarsal head and hallux. There was an inverse relationship for the hallux and first metatarsal head in that an increase in dorsiflexion angle of fusion increased pressure under the first metatarsal head and decreased pressure under the hallux. Peak pressure and pressure-time interval were minimized at 24.7° and 21.3° respectively.

Budhabhatti and colleagues,[40] in a finite element modeling of the first ray of the foot, found that each 1° change in dorsiflexion and valgus fixation angles in first MTPJ arthrodesis altered peak hallux pressure by 95 (9%) and 22 kPa (2%) respectively. With heel rise, the FHL imparts significant stress across the first MTPJ region.[41] Ankle immobilization may decrease forces across the first MTPJ by diminishing tendon variables. This approach may be more prudent with less stable fixation, but may also decrease blood flow.

With ankle motion, there is an increase in first metatarsal declination with heel-off during gait that can lead to increase stress across the first MTPJ.[42] Fixation must maintain bone apposition as well as resist forces about the first MTPJ associated with gait if limited weight bearing with ankle mobilization is allowed. Factors that affect bending moment, shear forces across the metatarsal, and axial load through the metatarsal are body weight, metatarsal declination, and length.[43] A forefoot cavus foot type in an obese individual with a long first metatarsal may have increased relative loads necessitating a stronger fixation construct and differing postoperative protocol than a rectus foot in a patient with a normal body mass index and normal metatarsal parabola. Standardization of postoperative protocol that allows ankle mobilization and heel weight bearing may need to consider these factors for individual patients.

VASCULAR SUPPLY

An understanding of the vascular network to the first ray is important to appreciate how varying dissection techniques may affect healing. Different fixation techniques can include varying amounts of soft tissue dissection about the first MTPJ. Dissection techniques by individual surgeons regardless of the fixation may also have an impact on healing potential and union rates. Over the decades there have been numerous studies documenting individual findings related to vascular supply to the first MTPJ.[44–49] Different preparation, dissection, and assessment techniques within these studies account for some of the differences in their findings.

There is a general consensus that the first metatarsal nutrient artery penetrates the lateral metatarsal in its middle third region. Some studies show it arising mainly from the first plantar metatarsal artery,[49] whereas others show it usually arising from the first dorsal metatarsal artery.[44,47] There are also different findings regarding the major region of pericapsular blood supply extending to the first metatarsal head.[44,46,47,49] Both the plantar-lateral and dorsomedial regions have been identified as the major plexus within the head region. These studies show that periosteal and capsular dissection has the potential to affect blood flow to the fusion site. There is little disagreement regarding plantar nutrient blood flow coming from the plantar surface into the midshaft region of the proximal phalanx.[44,45]

Crossed-screw fixation, K-wire fixation, and Steinman pins do not require additional soft tissue dissection beyond that required for joint surface preparation. Screw fixation directed from the medial aspect of the proximal phalanx and exiting the lateral metatarsal cortex provides the opportunity to disrupt the nutrient artery of the first metatarsal. Likewise, parallel screw fixation directed from the dorsal aspect of the metatarsal to the plantar aspect of the distal phalanx provides the opportunity to disrupt the nutrient vessel to the proximal phalanx. Conical reaming typically requires additional dissection, compared with planar resection, about the MTPJ capsular region. Many conical reamer systems use a guidewire, and to manipulate the bone segments to allow joint resection necessitates this increased dissection. In vivo studies and operative techniques that include images of reaming techniques show the severity of periosteal capsular stripping associated with this technique.[8,12] This type of stripping has not shown a clinically significant negative impact on fusion rate because it is commonly described in current in vivo studies with high union rates. However, it cannot be determined whether fusion rates would be higher with current fixation constructs with less dissection off the periosteal capsular surfaces. With severe fibrosis, as in revisional cases or previously operated sites, additional periosteal stripping may be required to allow manipulation of the joint surfaces for conical reaming devices. The periosteum is typically stripped away from the bone for plate fixation. Fixation that is not applied over the periosteal surface also requires additional periosteal stripping. Non–locking plate fixation applied directly over the periosteal capsular tissues could impede blood flow by virtue of the screws pulling the plate down toward the bone. Locking plates have the ability to be a more biologic fixation, if applied over the periosteum, but have a greater chance for adhesions to the extensor hallucis longus tendon because many plates contain some form of titanium. These adhesions could require eventual removal of the plate if the patient finds them uncomfortable. Multiple screws within plates of any kind have the opportunity to damage intramedullary blood flow, as does crossed-screw fixation more than K-wire fixation.

POSTOPERATIVE FOOT PROTECTION

There are many postoperative mobilization managements for first MTPJ arthrodesis.[24,50–52] Most studies currently either place patients in a surgical shoe or premade walking cast. Meek and Anderson[50] compared crepe dressings with plaster slipper casts, both protected by a cast shoe. There was no significant difference in union rate. Patients showed a more favorable procedure outlook in the crepe bandage group as well as returning to normal activity quicker. The plaster slipper casts allowed exposure of the hallux, permitting direct pressure on the hallux and retrograding stress across the first MTPJ. Fiberglass has now replaced plaster for slipper casts and it would be interesting to assess whether the more rigid material would provide a higher union rate in a similar study. It would also be of interest to discern what stress ending the cast proximal and distal to the hallux would impart.

Young and colleagues[24] compared different premade cast boots with fiberglass casts in a cadaveric study, testing their ability to protect a first MTPJ arthrodesis. The boot that provided the least flex in the ankle and the least movement of the foot and ankle within the boot performed the best. A description of how the fiberglass cast was applied was not provided.

Wu and colleagues[51] performed a study on the effects of the rocker sole and solid-ankle cushion-heel heel on kinematics in gait. Forefoot joint excursion across the first MTPJ in the sagittal plane with the rocker under the metatarsal area were significantly less than with flat-soled shoes during walking and ascending and descending stairs.

Budhabhatti and colleagues,[40] in their study on finite element modeling of the first ray to study design interventions, noted that insole material could reduce peak pressures under the hallux and first metatarsal head (Poron provided a reduction of peak pressures of 68% and 69%, respectively).

POSTOPERATIVE WEIGHT-BEARING STATUS

Investigators are intimately involved with their studies and, at times, forgo detailed information, not realizing how it affects critical review of their studies. When it comes to first MTPJ arthrodesis, immediate full postoperative weight bearing often means different things to different investigators. For some it means weight bearing on the heel and lateral aspect of the foot within a surgical shoe.[24] For others it means weight bearing in a below-the-knee walking cast,[53] and in others it may mean full forefoot load through the first ray segment during gait, including traversing stairs.[14,54] However, simple communication with an author can dispel an incorrect assumption.

When reviewing in vivo articles titled as weight bearing studies related to first MTPJ arthrodesis, it is hoped that, in addition to defining weight-bearing status, there has been some previous research to define the load applied to the first ray during gait with the apparatus described. Testing a single fixation construct is also preferred, with a large sample population that allows a power analysis to establish significance.

It has been estimated that 700 N of force can extend through the first MTPJ during gait in a 75-kg individual. There has been no strength or strain study that has shown a fixation construct to be able to withstand this amount of load without failure. It is unlikely that patients are unrestricted full weight bearing across the first MTPJ with today's appliances as footwear protection. One answer to improving fusion rates may not be in the fixation method but in the postsurgical apparatus worn. If the desire is to normalize gait as quickly as possible, a surgical shoe design with the following tenets may assist in this endeavor:

- Rocker sole positioned to specifically reduce ground reactive forces at the MTPJ region
- Low platform to avoid increasing stress to the hip
- Rigid shank or last to prevent bending moment across the first MTPJ
- Pliable stress-absorbing material on skin-shoe interface side of the last
- Buildup of material to make contact with the arch to prevent flattening of the medial column

Most surgeons have had patients experience hip pain or difficulties from heel-wedge shoes or various forms of walking boots. Although this is not related to fusion rate, it affects patient satisfaction and can lead to new disorders that require treatment.

COST

There are multiple variables involved in the cost-effectiveness of fixation for first MTPJ arthrodesis. Included in this list are the basic cost of the fixation construct, operating room costs, symptomatic nonunions that require revision, and costs associated with additional intervention if removal is needed. There have been no studies to show that there is 1 superior fixation device when it comes to rate of union. There are no studies that show a statistically significant quicker time to fusion between those constructs that achieve similarly high union rates. There are studies that show a cost benefit to use of crossed screws compared with specific plating systems taking into consideration some of the parameters discussed earlier.[15,55,56] When reviewing cost studies, it is preferable if a single surgeon performs all the cases with each type of fixation device trialed, which would provide better comparisons of how dissection time, joint preparation, and basic familiarity with the fixation influence operating room costs, including associated anesthesia and radiology expenses.

PATIENT COMPLIANCE

Patient compliance related to poor postoperative direction, lack of postoperative gait education, or lack of understanding by the patient leaves potential room for improvement in union rates for patients who inadvertently overload the first MTPJ. For patients allowed to weight bear in some capacity, it is preferred that the patient receives gait training before the procedure and that the gait trainer and patient are confident that the patient understands what is expected. Lasting anesthesia effects could affect this education process if gait training is performed after surgery. However, patients commonly associate pain with noncompliance and do not realize that they are repeatedly loading the fusion site in the absence of pain. Other patients disregard direction and weight bear as they desire.[57]

SUMMARY

The best fixation for first MTPJ arthrodesis is the method by which the individual surgeon obtains the best results. The postoperative protocol and protective shoe wear need to compliment the specific fixation technique. That requirement does not justify use of orthobiologics and fixation techniques that are exorbitant in cost. Cost control is a concern and an ethical responsibility. To use a construct that costs the hospital significantly more and provides no advantages or benefits compared with less expensive fixation methods is difficult to justify. However, ease of application is a significant advantage to justify use of a fixation technique. Not all surgeons find inserting 2 crossed screws quicker or easier than a dorsal plate and lag screw. Intraoperative complications from the insertion process could affect union rate, outcome, and overall expense, and this alone may justify the use of a more expensive product.

The literature allows clinicians to see fixation constructs and surgical techniques to which they may not normally be exposed. In vitro studies provide an opportunity for strength and strain studies to compare new technologies with the previous traditional standards.

Obtaining results similar to what some studies identify can involve a trial-and-error process. It is imperative that investigators detail every aspect of their process, not just the specific fixation, to allow others more closely to replicate it.

A careful review of the literature can provide a different assessment from what abstracts and conclusions of individual studies provide. Joint surface preparation, fixation technique, postoperative protocol, and protective shoe wear all affect outcome. The apparent concern within the literature for superiority of one joint preparation technique over another has yet to be proved of any clinical significance. The reviewed in vitro studies show a superiority of planar joint resection over current spherical reaming systems. However, misinterpretation of study details is common within the literature when citing outside references. The surgeon must take into consideration comorbidities, patient life situation, and cost when deciding what fixation to use. Surgeons are fortunate that there is not just 1 fixation technique available. Each surgeon should have a familiarity with several techniques that allows the one that is best for the individual patient to be chosen.

REFERENCES

1. Agoropoulos Z, Efstathopoulos N, Mataliotakis J, et al. Long-term results of first metatarsophalangeal joint fusion for severe hallux valgus deformity. Foot Ankle Surg 2001;7:9–13.

2. Santini AJ, Walker CR. First metatarsophalangeal joint fusion: a low profile plate technique. Foot Ankle Surg 2001;7:15–21.
3. Sharma V, Geary NP. Long term retrospective analysis of the first metatarsophalangeal joint arthrodesis with two crossed screws. Foot 2002;11:199–204.
4. Choudhary RK, Theruvil B, Taylor GR. First metatarsophalangeal joint arthrodesis: a new technique of internal fixation by using memory compression staples. J Foot Ankle Surg 2004;43(5):312–7.
5. Aslam N, Ribbans WJ. First metatarsophalangeal joint arthrodesis using a Vitallium plate with a mean two year follow up. Foot Ankle Surg 2005;11:197–201.
6. Brodsky JW, Passmore RN, Pollo FE, et al. Functional outcome of first metatarsophalangeal joint fusions using parallel screw fixation. Foot Ankle Int 2005; 26(2):140–6.
7. Patil S, Chojnowski A, Alber J. A retrospective analysis of first metatarsophalangeal joint fusions. Foot Ankle Surg 2005;11:113–6.
8. Goucher NR, Coughlin MJ. Hallux metatarsophalangeal joint arthrodesis using dome shaped reamers and dorsal plate fixation: a prospective study. Foot Ankle Int 2006;27(11):869–76.
9. Sharma H, Bhagat S, Deleeuw J, et al. In vivo comparison of screw versus plate and screw fixation for first metatarsophalangeal arthrodesis: does augmentation of internal compression screw fixation using a semi-tubular plate shorten time to critical and radiologic fusion of the first metatarsophalangeal joint (MTOJ)? The Foot 2002;11:199–204.
10. Grondal L, Stark A. Fusion of first metatarsophalangeal joint, a review of techniques and considerations presentation of our results in 22 cases. Foot 2008; 15:86–90.
11. Mah CD, Banks AS. Immediate weight bearing following first metatarsophalangeal joint fusion with Kirschner wire fixation. J Foot Ankle Surg 2009;48(1):3–8.
12. Patel A, Baumhauer J. First metatarsophalangeal joint arthrodesis. Oper Tech Orthop 2008;18:216–20.
13. Bennett GL, Sabetta J. First metatarsophalangeal joint arthrodesis: evaluation of plate and screw fixation. Foot Ankle Int 2009;30(8):752–7.
14. Wassink S, van den Oever M. Arthrodesis of first metatarsophalangeal joint using a single screw: retrospective analysis of 109 feet. J Foot Ankle Surg 2009; 48(6):653–61.
15. Kumar S, Prahanm R, Rosenfeld PF. First metatarsophalangeal arthrodesis using a dorsal plate and a compression screw. Foot Ankle Int 2010;31(9):797–801.
16. Bauer T, Jortat-Jacob A, Hardy P. First metatarsophalangeal joint percutaneous arthrodesis. Orthop Traumatol Surg Res 2010;96:567–73.
17. Besse JL, Choutteau J, Laptoiu D. Arthrodesis of the first metatarsophalangeal joint with ball and cup reamers and osteosynthesis with pure titanium staples radiological evaluation of a continuous series of 54 cases. Foot Ankle Surg 2010;16:32–7.
18. Sung W, Kluesner AJ, Irrgang J, et al. Radiographic outcomes following primary arthrodesis of the first metatarsophalangeal joint in hallux abductovalgus deformity. J Foot Ankle Surg 2010;49:446–51.
19. Hunt KJ, Ellington K, Anderson RB, et al. Locked versus nonlocked plate fixation for hallux MTP arthrodesis. Foot Ankle Int 2011;32(7):704–9.
20. Roukis TS, Meusnier T, Auguoyard M. Incidence of nonunion of the first metatarsophalangeal joint arthrodesis for severe hallux valgus using crossed, flexible titanium intramedullary nails and a dorsal static staple with immediate weight-bearing in femal patients. J Foot Ankle Surg 2012;51:433–6.

21. Hyer CF, Scott RT, Swiatek M. A retrospective comparison of four plate constructs for first metatarsophalangeal joint fusion: static plate, static plate with lag screw, locked plate, and locked plate with lag screw. J Foot Ankle Surg 2012;51:285–7.

22. Dening J, van Erve RH. Arthrodesis of the first metatarsophalangeal joint: a retrospective analysis of plate versus screw fixation. J Foot Ankle Surg 2012; 51:172–5.

23. Curtis MJ, Meyerson M, Jinnah RH, et al. Arthrodesis of the first metatarsophalangeal joint: a biomechanical study of internal fixation techniques. Foot Ankle 1991;14(7):395–9.

24. Young D, Stone NC, Molgaard J, et al. A biomechanical study in cadavers of cast boots used in early postoperative period after first metatarsophalangeal joint arthrodesis. Can J Surg 2003;46(3):183–6.

25. Sykes A, Hughes AW. A biomechanical study using cadaveric toes to test the stability of fixation techniques employed in arthrodesis of the first metatarsophalangeal joint. Foot Ankle 1986;7(1):18–25.

26. Rongstad KM, Miller GJ, Vander Griend RA, et al. A biomechanical comparison of four fixation methods of first metatarsophalangeal joint arthrodesis. Foot Ankle Int 1994;15(8):415–9.

27. Buranosky DJ, Taylor DT, Sage RA, et al. First metatarsophalangeal joint arthrodesis: quantitative mechanical testing of six-hole dorsal plate versus crossed screw fixation in cadaveric specimens. J Foot Ankle Surg 2001;40(4): 208–13.

28. Neufeld SK, Parks BG, Melamed EA, et al. Arthrodesis of the first metatarsophalangeal joint: a biomechanical study comparing memory compression staples, cannulated screws, and a dorsal plate. Foot Ankle Int 2002;23(2):97–101.

29. Molloy SM, Burkhart BG, Jasper LE, et al. Biomechanical comparison of two fixation methods for first metatarsophalangeal joint arthrodesis. Foot Ankle Int 2003;24(2):169–71.

30. Politi J, Hayes J, Njus G, et al. First metatarsophalangeal joint arthrodesis: a biomechanical assessment of stability. Foot Ankle Int 2003;24(4):332–7.

31. Faraj AA, Naraen A, Twigg P. A comparative study of wire fixation and screw fixation in arthrodesis for the correction of hallux rigidus using an in vitro biomechanical model. Foot Ankle Int 2007;28(1):89–91.

32. Müller ME, Allgower M, Schneider R, et al. Manual of internal fixation. Berlin: Springer-Verlag; 1970.

33. Singh B, Draeger R, Del Gaizo DJ, et al. Changes in length of first ray with two different first MTP fusion techniques: a cadaveric study. Foot Ankle Int 2008; 29(7):722–5.

34. Jung HG, Zaret DI, Park BG, et al. Effect of first metatarsal shortening and dorsiflexion osteotomies on forefoot plantar pressure in a cadaver model. Foot Ankle Int 2005;26(9):748–53.

35. Jacob HA. Forces acting in the forefoot during normal gait-an estimate. Clin Biomech 2001;16:783–92.

36. Beertema W, Draijer WF, van Os JJ, et al. A retrospective analysis of surgical treatment in patients with symptomatic hallux rigidus: long term follow up. J Foot Ankle Surg 2006;45(4):244–51.

37. Rittweger J. Ten years muscle-bone hypothesis: what have we learned so far? Almost a festschrift. Musculoskelet Neuronal Interact 2008;8(2):174–8.

38. Kirane YM, Michelson JD, Sharkey NA. Evidence of isometric function of flexor halluces longus muscle in normal gait. J Biomech 2008;41:1919–28.

39. Bayomy A, Aubin PA, Sangeorzan BJ, et al. Arthrodesis of the first metatarso-phalangeal joint: a robotic cadaver study of the dorsiflexion angle. J Bone Joint Surg Am 2010;92(8):1754–64.
40. Budhabhatti SP, Erdemir A, Petre M, et al. Finite element modeling of the first ray of the foot: a tool for the design of interventions. J Biomech Eng 2007;129:750–6.
41. Ferris L, Sharkey NA, Smith TS, et al. Influence of extrinsic plantar flexors on forefoot loading during heel rise. Foot Ankle Int 1995;16(8):464–73.
42. Kristen KH, Berger K, Kampla W, et al. The first metatarsal bone under loading conditions: a finite element analysis. Foot Ankle Clin North Am 2005;10:1–14.
43. Stokes AF, Hutton WC, Scott JRR. Forces acting in the metatarsals during normal walking. J Anat 1979;129:579–90.
44. Shereff MJ, Yang QM, Kumer FJ. Extraosseous and intraosseous arterial supply to first metatarsal and metatarsophalangeal joint. Foot Ankle 1987;8(2):81–93.
45. Vega M, Resnick D, Black JD, et al. The intrinsic and extrinsic arterial supply to the proximal phalanx of the hallux. Foot Ankle 1985;5(5):257–63.
46. Jones KJ, Feiwell LA, Freedman EL, et al. The effect of chevron osteotomy with lateral capsular release on the blood supply to the first metatarsal head. J Bone Joint Surg Am 1995;77(2):197–204.
47. Malal JJG, Shaw-Dunn J, Kumar CS. Blood supply to the first metatarsal head and vessels at risk with a chevron osteotomy. J Bone Joint Surg Am 2007;889(9):2018–22.
48. Alagoz MS, Orbay H, Usyal AC, et al. Vascular anatomy of the metatarsal bones and the interosseous muscles of the foot. J Plast Reconstr Aesthet Surg 2009;62:1227–32.
49. Rath B, Notermans HP, Franzen J, et al. The microvascular anatomy of the meta-tarsal bones: a plastination study. Surg Radiol Anat 2009;31:271–7.
50. Meek RMD, Anderson AG. Plaster versus crepe bandage after first metatarso-phalangeal joint fusion. Foot Ankle Surg 1998;4:213–7.
51. Wu WL, Rosenbaum D, Su FC. The effects of rocker sole and SACH heel on kinematics in gait. Med Eng Phys 2004;26:639–46.
52. Dayton P, McCall A. Early weightbearing after first metatarsophalangeal joint arthrodesis: a retrospective observational case analysis. J Foot Ankle Surg 2004;43(3):156–9.
53. Lampe HI, Fontijne P, van Linge B. Weight bearing after arthrodesis of the first metatarsophalangeal joint a randomized study of 61 cases. Acta Orthop Scand 1991;62(6):544–5.
54. Berlet GC, Hyer CF, Glover JP. A retrospective review of immediate weightbear-ing after first metatarsophalangeal joint arthrodesis. Foot Ankle Spec 2008;1(1):24–8.
55. Hyer CF, Glover JP, Berlet GC, et al. Cost comparison of crossed screws versus dorsal plate construct for first metatarsophalangeal joint arthrodesis. J Foot Ankle Surg 2008;47(1):13–8.
56. Watson AD, Kelikian AS. Cost-effectiveness comparison of three methods of in-ternal fixation for arthrodesis of the first metatarsophalangeal joint. Foot Ankle Int 1998;19(5):304–10.
57. Bennett GI, Kay DB, Sabatta J. First metatarsophalangeal joint arthrodesis: an evaluation of hardware failure. Foot Ankle Int 2005;26(8):593–6.

End-Stage Osteoarthritis of the Great Toe/Hallux Rigidus

A Review of the Alternatives to Arthrodesis: Implant Versus Osteotomies and Arthroplasty Techniques

Adam D. Perler, DPM[a,b,c,*], Victor Nwosu, DPM[b],
Drew Christie, DPM[c], Kellie Higgins, DPM[c]

KEYWORDS

- Hallux rigidus • Arthrodesis • Cheilectomy • Interpositional arthroplasty
- First metatarsophalangeal joint • Partial joint replacement • Hemiarthroplasty
- Total joint replacement

KEY POINTS

- Hallux rigidus is defined as end-staged arthrosis of the first metatarsophalangeal joint. Clinically, there is significant limitation and pain with range of motion of the joint. Radiographically, there is pronounced collapse of the joint space with subchondral sclerosis, extra-articular bone proliferation, and often cystic formation.
- Although the literature supports arthrodesis as being the gold standard for the treatment of end-staged hallux rigidus, there are several other treatments available that can either prolong the life of the remaining joint or artificially mimic the original biomechanics by replacing a portion of or the entire joint with the added advantage of preserving joint mobility.
- There are several new and emerging joint preservative techniques that may delay or prevent the need for a joint-destructive procedure, such as arthrodesis or arthroplasty.

Disclosure: Consultant, Product Development, Biomet, Warsaw, IN; Key Opinion Leader, Artimplant USA, Prosper, TX (A.D. Perler).
[a] Saint Vincent's Hospital System, Indianapolis, IN, USA; [b] American Health Network Reconstructive Foot and Ankle Surgical Fellowship, Indianapolis, IN, USA; [c] Foot and Ankle Residency Program, Saint Vincent's Hospital, Indianapolis, IN, USA
* Corresponding author. American Health Network, 1080 North Green Street, Suite 200, Brownsburg, IN 46112.
E-mail address: adperler@gmail.com

Clin Podiatr Med Surg 30 (2013) 351–395
http://dx.doi.org/10.1016/j.cpm.2013.04.011   **podiatric.theclinics.com**

INTRODUCTION

Hallux rigidus is one of the most common forms of degenerative joint disease of the foot and ankle and represents end-stage arthritis of the first metatarsophalangeal joint (MPJ).[1] If left untreated, hallux rigidus can cause significant pain and debilitation, which often leads to altered gait mechanics, decreased activity levels, and a marked reduction in patients' quality of life. Pain can occur directly from the degenerative joint changes, inflammation, and restriction in motion or can be secondary to adaptively favoring away from the arthritic joint. Although this condition has been well documented in the literature for more than a century, the ultimate treatment regimen has not been established and, therefore, remains a controversial topic. The literature clearly supports joint fusion as being one of the more predictable and reproducible treatments with satisfactory outcomes; however, there are reports of several motion-sparing alternatives that can either delay or prevent the need to sacrifice the intended motion of the joint.[1–3] This article focuses on exploring the motion-sparing alternatives to arthrodesis in the treatment of end-staged hallux rigidus. Ultimately, the real gold standard technique should be one that reliably restores normal foot function, eliminates pain, achieves good alignment and cosmesis, and significantly improves patients' quality of life both immediately and long term, while preserving future treatment options should the original plan fail.

DEFINITION OF HALLUX RIGIDUS

Hallux rigidus is a condition that leads to a reduction of sagittal plane range of motion of the first MPJ and was originally described by Nicoladoni[4] in 1881. Cotterill[5] introduced the term *hallux rigidus* in 1877. It is typically most painful on dorsiflexion excursion of the toe during the push-off phase of the gait cycle. Although it is most commonly caused by degenerative joint disease, it can also be linked to various other conditions, such as inflammatory arthropathies, osteoarthritis dissecans, or trauma to the articular surface or capsule of the first MPJ. The term *hallux limitus* has also been used to describe an earlier and less advanced phase of hallux rigidus with a painful limitation of dorsiflexion of the first MPJ.[6,7] As the joint goes through an arthritic breakdown over time, the body typically responds by laying down new bone to limit the overall excursion of the toe. The progression of arthritis is observed both radiographically and clinically as dorsal periarticular osteophytes form over the joint and act as a buttress in an attempt to limit motion, which, in turn, leads to mechanical impingement, further cartilage breakdown, osteolysis, and eventual ankylosis **(Fig. 1).**[8]

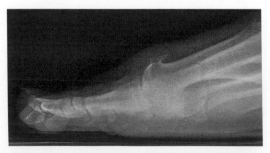

Fig. 1. Lateral radiograph with dorsal osteophytic formation and joint space narrowing.

CAUSE

The first MPJ is subjected to a significant amount of loading and stress throughout the gait cycle and during weight-bearing activities.[9] Normal first MPJ dorsiflexion during gait has been reported to range from 42° to 60°.[10] Over a lifetime, the joint can undergo the development of degenerative changes secondary to repetitive stresses. Osteoarthritis of the first MPJ has been reported to affect between 35% and 65% of adults older than 65 years.[11] Although unilateral presentations are most often secondary to traumatic causes,[12] 95% of cases seem to be bilateral with nearly two-thirds reporting a positive family history.[13] Coughlin and Shurnas[13] indicated in their extensive hallux rigidus demographics study that the mean age of the onset of symptoms was 43 years, the average age of surgical intervention was 50 years, and hallux rigidus seems to be more prevalent in women than men.

CLINICAL PRESENTATION

Patients typically present complaining of pain and stiffness of the great toe joint. The pain is usually noted during maximal range of motion of the joint as seen during the initial push-off phase of gait. Pain in the great toe joint can make activities such as walking up inclines, stairs, squatting, walking, or running more difficult as the arthritic condition progresses.[14] Patients may complain of symptoms across the forefoot, lateral to the great toe, often secondary to altered gait mechanics and favoring away from the faltering joint as they attempt to reduce the load to area.[15] On physical examination, the joint is more often than not tender dorsally. In the later stages of hallux rigidus, there is often exuberant osteophytic formation in the periarticular area (**Fig. 2**). Adaptive bone formation is most commonly palpated dorsally and can involve a compression neuritis of the dorsomedial cutaneous nerve.[16] Passive range of motion will usually cause pain at or near the end points of extreme dorsiflexion or plantar flexion. In the early stages of hallux limitus, the pain is often located at the dorsal aspect of the joint and becomes more diffuse as the arthritis progresses.[14] Pain at the midrange of motion is usually seen with more severe arthritis. Crepitus of the joint is often a sign of exposed areas of subchondral bone. It is important to note where in the range of motion the crepitus occurs because this can be suggestive of the staging of the cartilage degeneration and help to decipher between diffuse breakdown of the cartilage bed versus a localized and pinpoint osteochondral defect. Pain and crepitus at the midrange of motion is often associated with a severe grade of hallux rigidus and

A   B

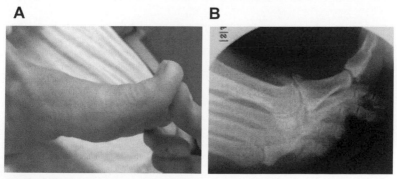

Fig. 2. (*A, B*) Clinical and radiographic findings on same patient with significant limitation of dorsiflexion of the first metatarsophalangeal joint secondary to exuberant dorsal osteophytic formation.

usually requires more extreme surgical measures, which may include joint-destructive procedures.[17]

RADIOGRAPHIC FINDINGS

The radiographic assessment of hallux limitus/rigidus should include weight-bearing anteroposterior (AP), lateral, and lateral oblique views of the foot. Advanced imaging modalities, such as magnetic resonance imaging (MRI) or computed tomography, are typically reserved for cases in which an osteochondral defect/lesion is to be ruled out. The joint spacing and metatarsal head shape should be evaluated on the AP views. Also, the density and integrity of the subchondral bone in the periarticular region including the sesamoids should be assessed. It should be noted that significant osteophytic formation dorsally can obstruct the view of the joint on the AP, therefore, giving the impression that the joint is further along the joint-destructive cycle than it may actually be. On the lateral view, the presence of joint-blocking osteophytes should be noted, along with the spacing of the joint and the overall biomechanical position of the entire first ray that may have contributed to faulty mechanical breakdown of the joint, absent any history of any traumatic events or the presence of systemic inflammatory arthropathy.

CLASSIFICATIONS

Several classification systems have been proposed in the literature to help guide the practitioner regarding correlating the severity of the clinical presentation with a potential treatment regimen. Although some of them do assist the practitioner with general treatment guidelines, none of them have truly linked the various stages of hallux limitus/rigidus to treatment based purely on a prognostic value or evidenced-based treatment regimen. The two most popular classification systems are the Regnauld classification system (**Table 1**) and the more comprehensive Coughlin and Shurnas classification system (**Table 2**). The inconsistency of the use of the classification systems in the literature has made it quite difficult to evaluate the outcomes of the various types of available hallux limitus/rigidus treatments (**Fig. 3**).[18]

TRADITIONAL CONSERVATIVE MANAGEMENT OF HALLUX RIGIDUS

Conservative measures should always be attempted before the discussion of surgical intervention, although the effectiveness of this pathway is significantly less beneficial

Table 1 Regnauld classification of hallux rigidus	
Grade	**Clinical Findings and Radiographic Findings**
1	Mild limitation of dorsiflexion and pain clinically; radiographically, mild dorsal spurring, mild subchondral sclerosis, and no sesamoid involvement
2	Broadening and flattening of the metatarsal head and proximal phalangeal base, focal joint space narrowing, structural first ray elevates, osteochondral defect, and/or sesamoid hypertrophy
3	Greater loss of joint space and near ankylosis, extensive osteophyte formation, osteochondral defects, extensive sesamoidal hypertrophy, with or without loose bodies

Data from Regnauld B. Disorders of the great toe. In: Elson R, editor. The foot: pathology, etiology, seminology, clinical investigation and treatment. New York: Springer-Verlang; 1986. p. 269–81.

Table 2
Coughlin and Shurnas' clinical and radiographic classification of hallux rigidus

Grade	Dorsiflexion	Radiographic Findings	Clinical Findings
0	40°–60°	Normal	No pain, only stiffness and some loss of motion
1	30°–40°	Dorsal osteophytes as main finding; minimal joint narrowing, flattening of the metatarsal head, and/or periarticular sclerosis	Mild and/or intermittent pain and stiffness at maximal dorsiflexion and/or plantar flexion of the joint
2	10°–30°	Periarticular osteophytes with mild to moderate joint narrowing, flattening of the metatarsal head, and/or periarticular sclerosis	Moderate to severe pain and stiffness with a more pronounced frequency; pain evoked near end range of motion of the joint
3	Less than or equal to 10°	Same as grade 2 but with the addition of cystic changes subchondrally and likely sesamoid irregularities	Nearly constant pain and stiffness with the pain being elicited with end range of motion, but not at midrange
4	Same as grade 3	Same as grade 3	Same as grade 3 but with pain present at midrange of passive motion of the joint

Data from Coughlin MJ, Shurnas PS. Hallux rigidus: grading and long-term results of operative treatment. J bone Joint Surg Am 2003;85:2702–88.

as the degenerative process of the great toe advances. From a medication viewpoint, nonsteroidal antiinflammatories as well as brief usage of oral steroids, such as methylprednisone, are aimed at reducing pain and inflammation but are not considered to be good long-term solutions because they do not typically alter the underlying cause of patients' pain. Topical prescriptive compound medications have the advantage of localized treatment with the ability to mix multiple medications, such as antiinflammatories with neuritic agents, and have been shown to be effective at addressing the symptoms of pain and swelling at the joint.[19] Shoe gear modifications, orthotic therapy with or without Morton extensions, and physical therapy are other well-documented conservative treatments of value; however, their value typically decreases as the deterioration of the joint progresses.[20]

Injection therapy is normally used as a diagnostic indicator; although it can have some therapeutic value, it is not typically seen as a long-term solution. Injection therapy can include the use of either corticosteroids or hyaluronic acid, although their long-term benefits are still not considered to be all that effective. Although corticosteroids can give temporary relief of pain, they do not modify the underlying cause of the arthritis and can have well-documented side effects, adversely affect the cartilage viability, and potentially retard the joint's ability to heal itself.[21] Also, one must use caution when using local anesthetics repetitively into a joint because there is evidence that intra-articular use of local anesthetics may have lasting detrimental effects on human articular cartilage and chondrocytes, especially at higher concentrations.[22] In one study, Pons and colleagues[23] compared the effectiveness of cortisone injections versus injectable nonsteroidal sodium hyaluronate for the treatment of pain and swelling associated with end-staged hallux rigidus. Interestingly enough, both groups of patients reported that their pain was significantly reduced at the 3-month follow-up; however, after 1 year approximately half of the patients in each group progressed on

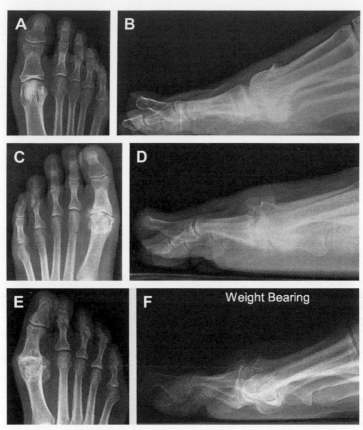

Fig. 3. (*A*) AP view demonstrating findings consistent with late grade I/early grade II Coughlin and Shurnas. (*B*) Lateral view demonstrating findings consistent with late grade I/grade II Coughlin and Shurnas. (*C*) AP view demonstrating findings consistent with grade III Coughlin and Shurnas. (*D*) Lateral view demonstrating findings consistent with grade III Coughlin and Shurnas. (*E*) AP view demonstrating findings consistent with grade IV Coughlin and Shurnas. (*F*) Lateral view demonstrating findings consistent with grade IV Coughlin and Shurnas.

to surgery. Although the use of hyaluronate-derived products has support in the knee, it is currently considered off-label for use in the foot. Also, some studies have demonstrated that it has favorable results compared with cortisone injections in the knee[24]; however, there is concern that, like cortisone, hyaluronic acid supplementation may actually accelerate the breakdown of cartilage.[25]

Another emerging conservative technique is the use of intra-articular injections autologous platelet-rich plasma (PRP). In a study that compares autologous PRP with nonsteroidal sodium hyaluronate injections of the knee, autologous PRP injections showed more and longer efficacy than Haluronic Acid (HA) injections in reducing pain and symptoms, and recovering articular function, especially for younger patients with early osteoarthritis or osteochondral lesions.[26] To date, PRP has not been seen to have the same potential of accelerated chondral breakdown and may actually improve the biologic repair of damaged cartilage and synovial tissues through the enhancement of anabolic reparative pathways and inhibition of catabolic processes associated with arthritis.[27] In vitro, PRP seems to potentiate chondrocyte proliferation, type II collagen, and proteoglycan formation.[28,29] Mesenchymal and amniotic fluid–derived stem stem cells are also being investigated for chondrocyte proliferation potential as another biologic adjunct cartilage regenerative medicine that may eventually be available for injection therapy.[30] This area will certainly be an area to watch over the next several years because minimally invasive orthobiologics and continued advancements in regenerative medicine could significantly shift the treatment paradigm for degenerative joint disease.

SURGICAL TREATMENTS OF HALLUX RIGIDUS: AN OVERVIEW

Once it has been established that conservative measures have failed to alleviate the patients' symptoms associated with hallux rigidus, surgical intervention is often the next step. It should be noted that in the current literature, there is no consensus on a clear surgical treatment algorithm for the treatment end-staged hallux rigidus. More often than not, each surgeon has preferences of treatments that they make available to their patients based on their own personal outcomes, training, and personal philosophy toward whether or not a lack of motion without pain using a joint-destroying fusion is an acceptable outcome versus an attempt to salvage motion, through the use of motion-sparing techniques that may require the need for future surgical intervention. Either way, each surgeon is ultimately faced with the ultimate task of selecting the surgical pathway that addresses each patient's specific set of pathophysiological factors and is based on the patient's realistic short-term and long-term expectations of their surgical outcomes and the understanding of the unique risks and benefits of the proposed techniques. Surgeons must also factor in their own tolerance of surgical risk, past outcomes/experience, training, and comfort levels with the types of procedures that think they can predictably execute.

The literature seems to favor cheilectomy with an excision of extra-articular spurring in the initial phases of osteoarthritis of the great toe.[31] Many individuals suggest that this is most effective if the cartilage wear pattern on the metatarsal head is located in the upper quarter of the joint surface (**Fig. 4**).[14,31–34] This procedure typically has a predictable outcome and more importantly leaves the joint intact, which keeps most future surgical options open should the joint continue to breakdown toward end-staged hallux rigidus. Depending on the causative factor, one should also assess if there are any contributing biomechanical issues that can be addressed at this stage, such as an elevated or elongated first ray, hallux valgus, pes planus, or ankle equinus. Addressing these at this point may prevent or prolong the further breakdown of the great toe joint. Interestingly enough and despite being regarded by many as the gold standard for the surgical treatment of an early staged hallux rigidus, there is about a 30% recurrence of dorsal osteophytes when treating with cheilectomy alone.[32] As the degenerative changes progress to include pain at the midway range of motion with continued collapse of the joint radiographically, the success rates of a cheilectomy diminish significantly.[17,32]

When treating the more advanced grades of hallux rigidus that have either failed a previous cheilectomy or would not likely benefit from a joint-preserving technique, the surgical treatment options should be tailored to fit the needs and expectations of each individual patient. The risks and benefits of each approach should be fully reviewed with each patient. Although the literature states that a successful fusion can often lead to a good surgical outcome, the concept of sacrificing motion to address a painful joint is not always the most appealing option for numerous patients, especially those who are young and active. It can also be said that surgical alternatives to fusion are constantly evolving, especially now that most orthopedic companies have identified the foot and ankle market as one of the fastest growing segments in orthopedic

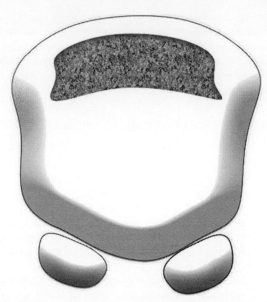

Fig. 4. The distal articular surface of the first metatarsal head as viewed distally with the cartilage wear pattern affecting the dorsal quarter surface.

business and are investing a great deal of money into research and development in the foot and ankle space. The other aspect of this is the more recent introduction/addition of regenerative medicine, which is really at its infancy stage of development but has great potential to open new doors to joint preservation through cellular cartilage regeneration. **Table 3** demonstrates the various possible treatment alternatives for progressing levels of hallux rigidus.

JOINT-PRESERVING PERIARTICULAR PROCEDURES

Joint preservation should always be the goal in the early phases of treating hallux rigidus, especially stages I, II, and early stage III. The key focus should be on restoring the mechanics of the joint and removing any excess bone that may interfere with normal joint function and rotation. The success of these procedures is quite dependent on the underlying condition of the articular cartilage. The following section reviews the most common periarticular procedures for early staged hallux rigidus.

Cheilectomy

The cheilectomy procedure is one whereby hypertrophic bone is removed from the dorsal one-third to one-quarter of the first metatarsal head (**Fig. 5**). In addition to this exostectomy, any proliferative bone is removed from the base of the proximal phalanx. A McGlamry elevator may be used to perform a plantar release of the soft tissues from the plantar aspect of the first MPJ.[35] The excess boney proliferation at the dorsal aspect of the joint consequently causes decreased dorsiflexor range of motion. Once these impeding factors or limitations have been removed, the end result is usually an increase in dorsiflexion excursion of the joint.

Although an exostectomy was suggested as early as 1927 at this location by Cochrane,[36] the first cheilectomy was not performed until more than 30 years later. Nilsonne[8] published a technique and his results in 1930; however, in 1959 DuVries[7] described in depth the cheilectomy procedure commonly recognized today. Although

Table 3
This table presents the treatment alternatives for progressing arthritic changes associated with hallux limitus/rigidus. The large arrow at the bottom of the chart represents the advancing arthritic changes and options from left to right (right being more advanced) and the smaller arrows within the chart represent the options that still potentially apply to the next level of advancing arthritic changes of the first MTPJ

Early-Stage Hallux Rigidus/Limitus (Grade I or II)	Mid-Stage Hallux Rigidus (Grade III) or Failure of Previous Cheilectomy	End-Stage Hallux Rigidus (Grade IV and/or Failure of Lesser Invasive Motion Sparing Technique)
Cheilectomy ± peri-articular decompressive osteotomy	**Joint-sparing techniques** • Peri-articular osteotomies • Interpositional grafting as a biologic spacer • Arthrodiastasis	**Joint-destructive procedures** *Motion-sparing techniques* • Hemi-implantation (resurfacing one side of the joint with a metallic-based technology) • Hemi-implantation with a secondary periarticular osteotomy • Hemi-biological (complete resurfacing one side joint with a biological barrier) • Total joint replacement
Chondral therapy If cartilage damage or OCD is present. • Microfracture (fibrocartilage stimulation) • Injection therapy (cortisone, viscosupplementation) • Chondral repair or replacement (hyaline cartilage restoration) • Orthobiological therapy (PRP, stem cell derived therapy)	**Chondral therapy** If cartilage damage to greater than the dorsal one-quarter quadrant of the metatarsal head or OCD is present	*Keller with/without interpositional arthroplasty* *Motion-sacrificing technique* • Great toe joint fusion
Advancing arthritic changes	**Joint-destructive procedures** *Functional motion-sparing techniques* • Hemi-implantation (resurfacing one side of the joint with a metallic-based technology) • Hemi-implantation with a secondary periarticular osteotomy • Hemi-biological (complete resurfacing one side joint with a biological barrier) • Total joint replacement *Keller with/without interpositional arthroplasty* *Motion-sacrificing technique* • Great toe joint fusion	

This table represents the various alternatives for the treatment of advancing degenerative changes.

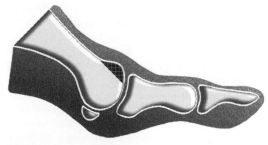

Fig. 5. Cheilectomy of the first metatarsal head.

modifications to the cheilectomy have been made, the basic principles of the procedure remain.

Multiple reviews have been completed on outcomes and results of the cheilectomy since the original report by DuVries in 1959. More recently in 2003, Coughlin and Shurnas[32] reported on results of 80 performed cheilectomy procedures, with a mean follow-up time period of 9.6 years. They found that 92% of these procedures were classified as successes, as evidenced by decreased pain and an increased range of motion and American Orthopedic Foot and Ankle Society's (AOFAS) scores. It should be noted that most of the procedures considered to be successes were as hallux limitus grades I and II preoperatively.

In 1997, Mackay and colleagues[31] reviewed and reported on outcomes based on preoperative grades of hallux limitus for 34 cases. In the end, satisfactory results of 94%, 100%, and 66% were accomplished for patients with grades I, II, and III, respectively. They concluded that the cheilectomy procedure was an excellent choice in surgical management of grades I and II hallux limitus.

In 2009, Lin and Murphy[37] reviewed 20 cheilectomy procedures that underwent a dorsal lateral approach over the lateral aspect of the first MPJ, as opposed to the standard approach. The investigators reported similar successful results as prior studies, with a 40% complication rate involving numbness at the first web space. They concluded that there was no specific advantage to the lateral approach versus the traditional approach.

Watermann-Green, 1927

The Watermann-Green procedure has evolved over the years from what was originally the Watermann. The original procedure, described in 1927, involved removing a dorsally based trapezoidal wedge from the proximal portion of the first metatarsal head.[38] The capital fragment and, thus, the articular cartilage is subsequently repositioned and appropriately fixated. Cavolo and colleagues[39] claimed that by removing the wedge and repositioning the cartilage, this procedure not only decreased the internal cubic content of the joint but also decompressed it. This decompression relaxes soft tissue attachments of the joint and allows for increased motion. Unfortunately, decreased stability exists because the osteotomy is made perpendicular to the shaft, not allowing for ideal fixation.[40] Because of the inherent instability of the capital fragment, a modification was made by removing a dorsally based triangular portion of bone from the same location.[41] This modification kept the plantar cortex and articular cartilage intact, while simultaneously offering mild decompression of the joint and protection of the sesamoids. The most recent modification is known as the Watermann-Green. This modification was a direct result of inadequate joint decompression of prior procedure modifications and was devised for more progressive cases of the condition.[42]

This procedural modification involves initially performing a dorsal cheilectomy, followed by a double arm osteotomy at the metatarsal head. The dorsal cut is parallel to the sagittal plane axis of the metatarsal, whereas the plantar cut is parallel to the weight-bearing surface of the metatarsal. A small section of bone is removed just proximal to the dorsal arm to allow for metatarsal shortening and, thus, decompression of the first MPJ. After all osteotomies have been made, fixation is recommended. Depending on how the osteotomies are oriented, this procedure can also allow for mild plantar flexion as well as correction of the proximal articular set angle (PASA).[43] In addition to the excess boney proliferation at the dorsal aspect of the joint, an elevated or elongated first metatarsal may be present. Although the concomitant cheilectomy improves previously restricted dorsiflexion, the double arm osteotomy accounts for the problematic metatarsal resulting in shortening and plantar flexion of the metatarsal head.

Dickerson and colleagues[44] reviewed 40 Watermann-Green procedures at a 4-year average follow-up. The investigators found satisfaction with 94% of patients relating their first MTPJ pain as greatly reduced.

Youngswick

The Youngswick procedure is a modification of the Austin osteotomy. Similar to the Austin, whereby 2 osteotomies are made and oriented 60° to one another at the metatarsal head, the Youngswick removes a small section of bone just proximal to the dorsal arm (**Fig. 6**).[45] Following the removal of any excess boney proliferation at the dorsal aspect of the joint, an elevated or elongated first metatarsal may remain. This double arm osteotomy is used to address an elongated and problematic metatarsal and results in shortening the metatarsal and plantar flexing the metatarsal head. The recommended fixation is similar to the Austin with desired positioning and can be achieved with one point of fixation because of the stability of the osteotomy.

Since the original description in 1982, the Youngswick has become a mainstay in surgical management of the condition (Youngswick 1982). Similar in some aspects to the Watermann-Green, the Youngswick has additional stability, which lends to its popularity. In 2007, Radovic and colleagues[46] described a modification to the Youngswick procedure to reduce the amount of metatarsal shortening, yet allow for greater ability to plantar flex the metatarsal. In this modification, the portion of bone removed from the dorsal arm of the osteotomy is inserted as a graft into the plantar arm of the osteotomy. This finding is consistent with a study in 2001 by Gerbert and colleagues,[47] who came to the conclusion that "the amount of plantar displacement is dependent upon the angle of the plantar arm."

Kessel-Bonney, 1958

The Kessel-Bonney procedure is one whereby a dorsally based wedge of bone is resected from the base of the proximal phalanx of the hallux.[48] The base of the proximal phalanx is left intact as the wedge is resected just distal to it (**Fig. 7**). An Akin osteotomy can be combined with this procedure for any additional valgus correction.[49] This procedure helps to reorient the hallux from a plantar flexed position, to a more dorsiflex position, on the metatarsal. Although this osteotomy does not allow

A

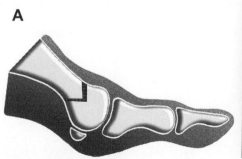

B

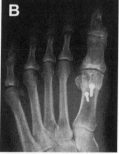

Fig. 6. (*A*) Decompression osteotomy (Youngswick modification) whereby a larger wedge of bone is removed from the dorsal cut to shift the articular surface of the metatarsal head proximal and plantar. (*B*) Five-year radiographic follow-up on a decompression Youngswick osteotomy for moderate grade hallux rigidus. Patient related little to no pain in the joint, despite the progressive joint space narrowing and subchondral cystic formation seen here.

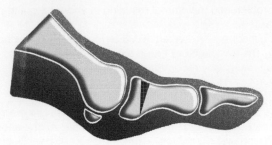

Fig. 7. Dorsal closing-wedge decompression osteotomy of the base of the proximal phalanx of the great toe (Bonney/Kessel procedure).

for increased dorsiflex range of motion of the first MPJ, it does create more dorsiflexion during functional gait at the level of the hallux. Although this procedure allows for increased functional dorsiflexion, it does not disturb the first MPJ capsule or weight-bearing tissues of the first metatarsal.[50]

Bonney and Macnab[51] initially described the procedure in 1952; however, it was not until 1958 that Bonney and Kessel[18] reported the results of their procedures. They initially devised the procedure in an effort to find an alternative to the joint-destructive Keller for the condition. Kilmartin, at an average follow-up of 29 months, evaluated 49 patients having undergone phalangeal osteotomy, producing results of 65% completely satisfied, 24% moderately satisfied, and 11% dissatisfied in 2005.[50] Additional studies have had success using the Kessel-Bonney as an adjunctive procedure with a cheilectomy. In 2008, Waizy and colleagues[34] completed a prospective study with 60 patients at an average follow-up time of 8 years, which found that the patients receiving the cheilectomy were 67% completely satisfied or satisfied and patients receiving the cheilectomy and Kessel-Bonney were 86% completely satisfied or satisfied.

Distal Oblique Osteotomy (Weil/Mau)

Although this procedure is most commonly associated with lesser metatarsals for shortening or decompression, it can also be used in the treatment of hallux limitus.[52] A single osteotomy is made, oriented dorsal distal to plantar proximal in the transverse plane, just proximal to the dorsal aspect of the articular cartilage of the metatarsal head. The angle of the osteotomy varies from 35° to 45°, which is somewhat larger than the traditional procedure used on lesser metatarsals (**Fig. 8**).[52] Two points of fixation are recommended for a more stable construct. This procedure addresses

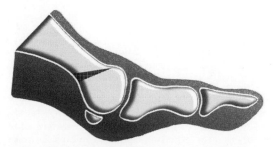

Fig. 8. Distal oblique osteotomy (Weil/Mau) of the metatarsal head with the ability to shift the distal articular surface inferior and proximal.

the condition at the metatarsal level, aiding in decompression of the joint by shortening the metatarsal and/or plantar flexing it. The degree of osteotomy made determines the amount of correction desired, whether shortening and/or plantar flexing,[52] resulting in increased dorsiflexor range of motion at the joint. The capital fragment can also be shifted medial or lateral to adjust for mildly elevated intermetatarsal angles.

In 2000, Ronconi and colleagues[52] had success in their study of 26 patients who received cheilectomy and Weil procedures, with 86% good to excellent outcomes. In 2006, LaMar and colleagues,[53] using bone models, completed a mechanical comparison and "found no statistically significant difference in strength between the Youngswick and the Weil"[53] using one point of fixation.

Drago (Double Metatarsal Osteotomy)

The Drago procedure is a combination or double metatarsal osteotomy. One osteotomy is a proximal metatarsal plantarflexing wedge osteotomy. Although this osteotomy places the metatarsal in a plantar flexed position, it also places the articular cartilage in a plantar flexed position. The other osteotomy is a modified Watermann osteotomy, which counteracts the plantar flexed articular cartilage of the already plantar flexed metatarsal.[54] Fixation is advised across the plantarflexory wedge osteotomy. Fixation is also recommended across the Watermann for additional stability; however, it is not required.

This double osteotomy addresses multiple issues of hallux limitus. As previously mentioned, the modified Watermann serves primarily to decompress the joint. Although the plantarflexory wedge osteotomy also offers decompression of the joint, its primary function is to plantar flex the metatarsal, allowing greater dorsiflexion at the first metatarsophalengeal Joint (MTPJ).

Sagittal Plane Z/Scarf

The sagittal Z or sagittal scarf procedure encompasses 3 arms. The distal arm spans and exits the lateral half of the metatarsal diaphysis, whereas the proximal arm spans and exits the medial half of the metatarsal diaphysis. The central arm is oriented in the longitudinal length of the midshaft (Fig. 9).[41] All osteotomies are made perpendicular to the weight-bearing surface. Two points of fixation are required for a stable construct. To shorten the metatarsal, a section of bone is removed just proximal to the distal arm and just distal to the proximal arm. To lengthen the metatarsal, simply move the capital fragment distally to the desired length. Gapping does occur with lengthening, yet grafting is not typically required.[55] Additional fixation is required should any type of grafting be implemented. With all osteotomies made perpendicular to the weight-bearing surface, this allows for plantar flexion of the capital fragment via rotation and transposition.[41] In addition, this procedure allows for shortening or lengthening for decompression or repositioning of the first MTPJ.

McGlamary and Banks[55] originally described the sagittal Z procedure in 1995. In 1996, Chang[33] obtained 86% good results with 32 cases of the sagittal Z procedure. In 1998, Viegas[56] followed 11 patients undergoing the same procedure and similarly obtained good to excellent outcomes from all procedures.

Lapidus Fusion

The Lapidus procedure is a procedure typically thought of for cases of hypermobility and severely increased intermetatarsal angles. The procedure we know as Lapidus today was initially described by Albrecht in 1911.[57] However, Lapidus[57] had not published his initial report on techniques until 1934, and the procedure became more widespread as a result.

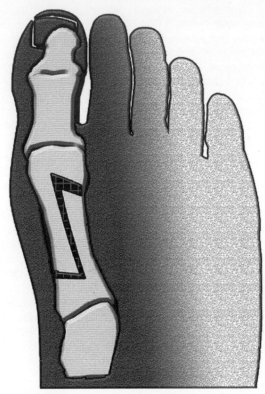

Fig. 9. Sagittal plane Z/scarf decompression first metatarsal osteotomy with ability to plantar flex and decompress the distal articular surface.

Although commonly used for hypermobile cases of hallux abducto valgus, this procedure can also be used for treatment of hallux limitus.[57] The procedure itself involves the removal of any excess boney proliferation about the metatarsal head. The first metatarsal and medial cuneiform articular surfaces are then denuded of cartilage to the level of subchondral bone with curettage, wedge resection, or reciprocal planing. The subchondral plate is then fenestrated to promote bleeding into the fusion site. Concerning hallux limitus, the metatarsal is translated inferiorly or plantarflexed through the first metatarsal-cuneiform joint, which helps to accommodate for shortening because of the longer lever arm (**Fig. 10**).[57] This joint is then fused using any number of acceptable fixations, based on physician preferences.

This proximal metatarsal osteotomy addresses multiple issues of hallux limitus, specifically elevation, elongation, and decompression. All of these concerns are addressed by the wedge resection at the first metatarsal–medial cuneiform joint. Once removed, the metatarsal can be plantar flexed and shortened accordingly. The remodeling of the dorsal or medial aspects of the metatarsal head serves as an adjunct cheilectomy to increase end dorsiflexor range of motion.[57]

Sagittal V

The sagittal V procedure is one whereby a V-shaped portion of bone is removed from the metatarsal neck or just proximal to the head. The osteotomy is oriented in the

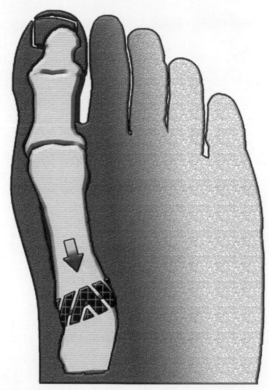

Fig. 10. Lapidus fusion of the first metatarsal/cuneiform joint can allow for decompression and plantar flexion of the distal articular surface of the first metatarsal. The arrow is representative of the compression achieved at the first metatarsal/cuneiform joint achieved with the Lapidus and the relative shortening of the first metatarsal allowing for decompression of the first MTPJ.

sagittal plane, with apex distally, angled from 45° to 55° (**Fig. 11**).[53] The capital fragment, depending on the angle of the osteotomy compared with the weight-bearing surface, is then manipulated to allow for shortening, plantar flexion, or both and then fixated.[58] With the removal of the V-shaped portion of bone, this procedure allows for decompression of the first MPJ by shortening the metatarsal. Because of the physicians' preference based on patients' needs, the osteotomy can be angled in the dorsal-distal to plantar-proximal direction[58] allowing the capital fragment to be manipulated to allow for decompression and/or plantar flexion.

LaMar and colleagues[53] attempted to test the mechanical loads and strength of 3 osteotomies, including Youngswick, sagittal V, and Weil. It was found "that the sagittal V osteotomy was significantly weaker and less stiff."[53] Because of concerns for the overall stability of the procedure, Robinson and Frank[58] described a modification of the procedure in 2005 known as the long arm decompression osteotomy. This procedure is similar to the sagittal V, with the apex distally and osteotomies in the sagittal plane, yet with a longer medial arm of the osteotomy. This modification allows for suggested increased decompression and plantar flexion from the original procedure, with increased stability and greater surface available for fixation.

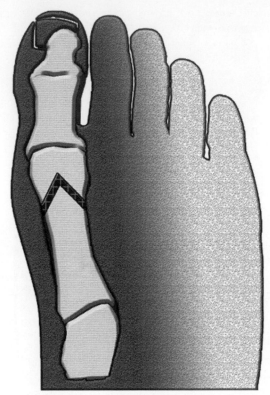

Fig. 11. The sagittal V is a distal metatarsal osteotomy that allows for decompression and plantar flexion of the distal articular surface of the first metatarsal.

The Moberg Procedure

The Moberg procedure[59] is a technique whereby a dorsal wedge of bone is resected from the base of the proximal phalanx of the hallux, just distal to it (**Fig. 12**). Two drill holes are placed in the base of the proximal phalanx on both sides of the osteotomy. Monofilament wire is then placed through the holes to close down the osteotomy. The Moberg procedure is typically reserved for patients with limited extension and more than enough flexion at the first MPJ.[59] Much like the Kessel-Bonney, the Moberg helps

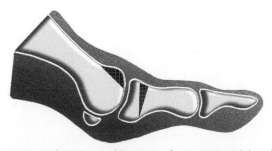

Fig. 12. The Moberg procedure is combination of a metatarsal head cheilectomy and closing-wedge decompression osteotomy of the proximal phalangeal base.

to reorient the hallux to a more dorsiflexed position on the metatarsal. Although this osteotomy does not allow for increased dorsiflexor range of motion of the first MTPJ, it does create more dorsiflexion during functional gait at the level of the hallux. Moberg published his report and techniques on 8 adult patients in 1979. Although it had a small sample size and short-term follow-up, he fails to report any complications. The longest follow-up at the time of the report was 5 years without complications and "good function" on outcome.[59]

Arthrodiastasis

Aldegheri and colleagues[60] coined the term *arthrodiastasis* and used it to describe extra-articular distraction of the hip joint. It uses the principle of ligamentotaxis to offload the articular surfaces of the joint and seems to provide an environment that is conducive for healing. This treatment is predicated on the knowledge that degenerative cartilage is capable of repair. Since that time, several studies have demonstrated that this technique can be useful for both ankle and first metatarsophalangeal applications.[61–64] The reparative capacity of the first metatarsophalangeal articular cartilage is enhanced through the mechanical offloading of the joint and maintenance of intra-articular synovial fluid pressure changes.[1]

Arthrodiastasis of the first MPJ can be used as a salvage procedure for a failed motion-sparing procedure or an alternative to or prolong the need for joint destructive procedures. Indications for arthrodiastasis of the first MPJ have been recommended to include a congruent joint but painful joint with reduced mobility, and moderate to severe arthritic changes.[1,64] The procedure involves the use of either a hinged or fixed

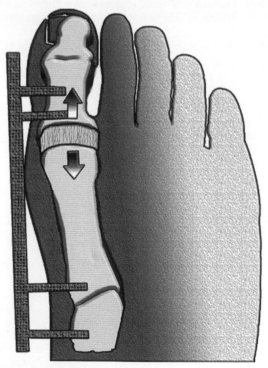

Fig. 13. Arthrodiastasis with the use of a monorail mini-external fixator to distract the articular surfaces away from each other and stretch/relax that soft-tissue around the first MPJ.

mini external fixator to obtain distraction and can be done in conjunction with other periarticular procedures, such as a cheilectomy, cartilage restoration or microfracture, or decompression and/or realignment osteotomy of the first MPJ (**Fig. 13**).[63,64]

Joint distraction has been shown to be a viable short-term option for joint preservation for moderate to early end-staged hallux rigidus. In a retrospective study by Abraham and colleagues,[64] the evaluation of the clinical and radiographic results associated with the treatment of hallux rigidus using the joint distraction with a hinged fixator for 2 months was described. Of the 10 distractions performed, radiographic examination revealed an increase in the joint space from 0.90 mm ± 0.70 mm preoperatively to 1.45 mm ± 0.44 mm postoperatively. The investigators also noted a significant improvement in the reported pain scores from a mean of 8.2 out of 10.0 preoperatively to 0.83 postoperatively.

BIOLOGIC INTERPOSITIONAL GRAFTING FOR HALLUX RIGIDUS

IA for the treatment of advancing hallux limitus is an intriguing option and continues to evolve as a viable alternative to fusion in certain candidates. Once it has been determined that arthritic breakdown of the joint exceeds the limitations of a dorsal cheilectomy (**Fig. 14**), regenerative cartilage strategies, and/or periarticular osteotomies, IA by means of a partial or total implant or a biologic spacer is usually next in line. Both treatments are general categories with varying levels of success; but techniques, rationale, and implantation techniques are constantly evolving with a better understanding of the true biomechanics of the great toe joint and its influence on the overall function the foot. As it stands, for most surgeons, providing these surgical options to their patients is primarily based on their own personal experiences with implantation, training, and philosophy. Although no one can argue that fusion has an extremely high success rate as documented in the literature,[32] the ultimate goal should be to relieve pain and restore proper biomechanics and functionality to the first MPJ. The only issue with this is that there are compromises no matter which direction one heads in decisionwise. Although a well-positioned and healed fusion is great at achieving pain relief and is much more predictable in the long run, it comes at the expense of eliminating motion, function, and positional adaptability of the joint. On the other hand, motion-sparing implantation procedures aim to restore motion and relieve pain but may be much less predictable in the long run and present unique challenges when it comes to surgical revision and salvage.[1,15] With this in mind, as the idea of interpositional

A   **B**

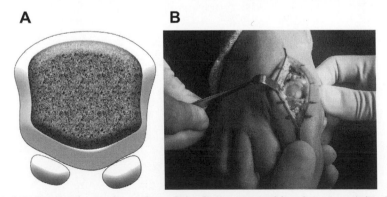

Fig. 14. (*A*) The distal articular surface of the first metatarsal head as viewed distally with the cartilage wear pattern affecting most of the joint surface. (*B*) Intraoperative demonstration of extreme cartilage wear on the metatarsal articular surface.

grafting matures as an emerging surgical option for hallux rigidus, there seems to be greater emphasis placed on the resection of less bone in the attempt to restore normal joint mechanics and function to keep as many options available should this step fail. Judicial restoration of joint function while preserving future options is especially more important to younger and more active patients.

RESECTION-BASED BIOLOGIC INTERPOSITIONAL ARTHROPLASTY

Interpositional arthroplasty (IA) for hallux rigidus is not a new concept and was originally described as an enhancement of the modified Keller arthroplasty with less bone resection and interposition of the dorsal MPJ capsule and extensor hallucis brevis tendon that act as a joint spacer to maintain length and overall position of the joint (**Fig. 15**).[65] Although this modification seems to have improved the predictability of this joint-destructive and motion-sparing procedure, there was still concern that a significant amount of patients at 1 year following the operation complained of weakness of the great toe at push-off (up to 72%), with transfer of pressure to the lesser MPJ often leading to metatarsalgia.[66] It was thought that this result was caused by the resection of the portion of the proximal phalangeal base and disruption of the insertion of the flexor hallucis brevis. To address this shortcoming, Mroczek and Miller[67] recommended the preservation of the flexor hallucis brevis by obliquely angling the proximal phalangeal cut to exit proximally just superior to the proximal phalangeal base (**Fig. 16**). This procedure also included a dorsal cheilectomy of the metatarsal head and a capsular interpositional arthroplasty. Kennedy and colleagues[68] also reported favorable outcomes (89% of patients reporting that they had little to no pain at the 1-year follow-up) using this modification. Using the same technique, Mackey and colleagues[69] compared IA with fusion and found that the IA group had higher AOFAS scores postoperatively (89.6% vs 64.5%, $P = .006$) at the 5.3-year follow-up. Even with these modifications, Keller procedures are still only recommended as an alternative to fusion in patients aged greater than 70 years and are less active when a shorter and less complex recovery is desired.[15]

ALTERNATIVE INTRA-ARTICULAR IA TECHNIQUES

The use of IA techniques along with minimal bone resection has continued to evolve away from initial Keller modifications. There is now emphasis on maintaining as much length of the joint as possible to keep all future avenues for surgical reconstruction, such as fusion or metallic resurfacing implants. Roukis and colleagues[70] have

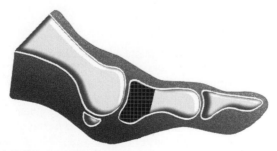

Fig. 15. Traditional Keller resectional arthroplasty involving the removal of the proximal one-third of the proximal phalanx. Recent modifications suggest using biologic spacer in attempt to prevent a dorsiflexion deformity of the hallux.

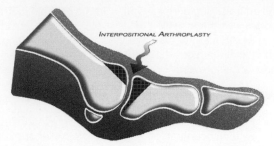

Fig. 16. Keller modification whereby an oblique resection of the proximal phalangeal base is performed, leaving the proximal and inferior portion intact to preserve the function of the flexor halluces brevis. This modification can also be combined with a metatarsal head cheilectomy and biologic interpositional arthroplasty.

suggested success with a similar capsular advancement technique with an intra-articular incorporation of a denervated capsule and periosteum flap. They thought the denervation of the interposed capsule/periosteal flap was key in preventing a painful joint secondary to symptomatic capsular impingement. Avoidance of symptomatic localized capsular impingement may also have been a key to the movement toward using alterative biologic spacers such a free autograft gracilis tendon bundle as suggested by Coughlin and Shurnas.[71] Although they and other investigators using similar autograft interpositional techniques reported good success, (**Tables 4** and **5**) this route does require use of a second surgical site. To avoid the increased morbidity of a secondary surgical site harvest of an autograft, Givissis and colleagues[72] reported on the successful use of allograft fascia lata. Berlet and colleagues[73] also introduced a minimal resection technique and the use of allograft regenerative tissue matrix cap laid over a lightly reamed metatarsal head with good initial results (**Fig. 17**). Finally, Heller and Robinson[74] suggested the use of Gelfoam (Pharmacia & Upjohn Co, Division of Pfizer Inc, New York, NY) as an interpositional spacer following microfracture of the involved areas of cartilage wear as a cheaper alternative to the aforementioned techniques. They deduced that this may act to stabilize the clot at the microfracture site and aid in the stimulation of fibrocartilage growth. They also suggested that this can be combined with periarticular decompression techniques or cheilectomy when microfracture techniques are used. They also suggested that they favored this method as an initial intervention, especially because it has little to no impact on the structural integrity of the periarticular bone, leaving all advanced future options on the table, including the use of other biologic interpositional spacers.

CHONDRAL RESTORATION AND REPAIR

Osteoarthritis is the process of when a joint undergoes degeneration of the chondral integrity and a breakdown of the subchondral bone. When osteoarthritis affects the great toe, there is usually the presence of osteochondral lesions and/or defects induced by either a traumatic event or repetitive localized stresses. Although most of the previously described surgical techniques for hallux rigidus, aside from fusion, focus on a mechanical decompression or synthetic resurfacing of the diseased articular surfaces, the idea of restoring and/or repairing the chondral surface has been always been intriguing. As orthrobiologics space has exponentially expanded in the last several years, there are now more and more chondral repair/restoration options available.

Table 4
Chart summarizes the various reported outcomes utilizing an inter-positional arthroplasty approach to resurfacing the first MTPJ

Graft Category	Study	Resection Method	IA Graft Details	Grade Mean f/u (mo) No. of Cases	Potential Benefits	Results (Percent of Good to Excellent)
IA Autograft	Lau & Daniels,[66] 2001 (comparative study)	Cheilectomy vs modified Keller with IA	EHB interposition	H&J II, III 24 mo 11 cases	↑ stability of Keller resectional arthroplasty	Cheilectomy: 78.0% EHB-IA: 72.0%
	Schenk,[123] et al (comparative study)	Traditional Keller vs modified Keller with IA	EHB interposition	H&J II, III 16.5 mo 14 cases	↑ stability of Keller resectional arthroplasty	89.0%
	Hamilton & Hubbard[124]	25% of proximal phalanx- modified Keller	EHB tenotomy Dorsal capsule sutured to the flexors	C&S III 37 cases	Prevents a dorsiflexion deformity of the hallux	94.0%
	Ozan,[125] et al	One-third base of proximal phalanx- modified Keller	EHB interposition with capsule Retrograde Kirschner-wire fixation/distraction	C&S III, IV 21 mo 19 cases	Aggressive decompression of the joint; however, reported ↓stability	84.2%
	Coughlin & Shurnas,[71] 2003	Reamed the base of the proximal phalanx to maintain plantar attachments	Free autograft gracilis tendon rolled into a 1.5 × 1.5 cm ball	C&S IV 42 mo 7 cases	Biologic spacer with maintenance of the length of the toe	86.0%
	Mackey et al,[69] 2010 (comparative study)	Fusion vs oblique cut Keller with preservation if the inferior proximal phalanx soft tissue attachments	Dorsal capsular interposition	End-staged hallux rigidus 63+ mo 10 modified Keller 12 fusions	Found good efficacy of their technique compared with their fusion group	AOFAS score Arthroplasty: 89.5 Fusion: 64.8

Abbreviations: ↑, increased; AOFAS Score, AOFAS Hallux; C&S, Coughlin and Shurnas hallux rigidus classification system; EHB, extensor halluces brevis; f/u, follow-up; H&J, Hattrup and Johnson hallux rigidus classification system[126]; MTP, IP Scale.

Table 5
This table represents the reported outcomes of interpostional arthroplasty techniques of the first MTPJ which utilize interposing allograft tissue

Graft Category	Study	Resection Method	IA Graft Details	Grade Mean f/u (mo) No. of Cases	Potential Benefits	Results (Percent of Good to Excellent)
IA Allograft	Hyer,[127] et al	Cartilage is reamed from the head of the metatarsal and the proximal phalanx is reamed obliquely	Regenerative tissue matrix graft	C&S III 64 mo 6 cases	Minimal bone resection; no secondary donor surgical site; easy revision if necessary	100% AOFAS Score Preoperative: 38 Postoperative: 65.8
	Heller & Robinson,[74] 2011	Only diseased cartilage is removed, followed by microfracture of the involved area	Gelfoam (absorbable gelatin powder; Pharmacia & Upjohn Co, Division of Pfizer Inc, New York, NY)	C&S III, IV 55 mo 30 cases	Cheap alternative to other allogenic grafts and nominal resection; may stabilize clotting at microfracture site for greater fibrocartilage repair rate	64.5% AOFAS Score Preoperative: 35 Postoperative: 74
	DeLaCruz,[128] et al	Aggressive dorsal wedge 10-mm total resection at MTP leaving plantar attachments intact	Allogenic cadaver meniscus shaped into a tortellini	H&J III 16.46 mo 13 cases	Minimal resection will not burn bridges to future treatment, such as fusion	AOFAS Score Preoperative: 52.54 Postoperative: 90.01

Abbreviations: AOFAS Score, AOFAS Hallux; C&S, Coughlin and Shurnas hallux rigicus classification; f/u, follow-up; H&J, Hattrup and Johnson hallux rigidus classification system.[126]

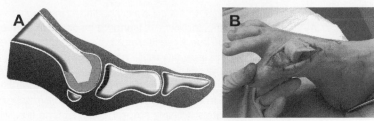

Fig. 17. (*A*) Minimal resection technique and the use of allograft regenerative tissue matrix cap laid over a lightly reamed metatarsal head. (*B*) Intraoperative picture demonstrating the minimal resection technique and the use allograft regenerative tissue matrix cap laid over a lightly reamed metatarsal head. (*Courtesy of* Terry M Philbin, DO, Orthopedic Foot and Ankle Center, Columbus, OH.)

MICROFRACTURE- CHONDRAL STIMULATION TECHNIQUES

Microfracture with stimulation of fibrocartilage growth as a patch has been recognized in the literature as a cost-effective but often temporary solution in an initial attempt to restore the integrity of a deteriorating articular surface.[75] Marrow-stimulation techniques using microfracture of the subchondral bone induces fibrin clot formation in the area of the chondral defect (**Fig. 18**). This clot contains pluripotent, marrow-derived mesenchymal stem cells, which are able to differentiate into fibrochondrocytes, resulting in a fibrocartilage repair with varying amounts of type I, II, and III collagen content.[76] Although some investigators report good long-term results with the use of microfracture techniques for cartilage defects, others suggest that the replacement fibrocartilage patch is more of a short-term solution that delays the

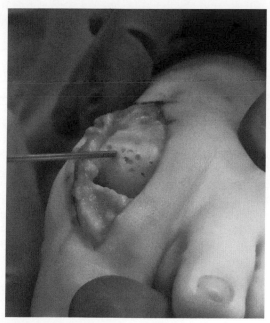

Fig. 18. Intraoperative example of microfracture of the degenerated articular surface of the first metatarsal head.

eventual breakdown of the joint and that its success may be linked inversely to the patients' age, activity level, and body mass index.[77–79] It should be noted that most of the research on microfracture is based on the knee literature, and very few studies have been done in relation to the great toe. Recently, there has been reported success using an arthroscopic approach to lesions of the first metatarsal head with spur removal and microfracture as safe and effective first-line treatment in the early stage of osteochondral defects of the great toe.[80,81] In the authors' experience, microfracture seems to be more effective in younger patients with early staged arthritis of the first MPJ and is typically performed using an open technique in conjunction with either cheilectomy and/or decompressive periarticular osteotomies of either the first metatarsal and/or proximal phalangeal base.

CHONDRAL REPAIR OR REPLACEMENT (HYALINE CARTILAGE RESTORATION)

The properties of native hyaline cartilage are amazingly complex and vital to the biomechanical health and function of a joint, especially the great toe. Articular cartilage damage is a persistent and increasing problem with the aging population, and treatments to achieve biologic repair or restoration of hyaline cartilage remains a challenge. Although the fibrocartilage stimulation via microfracture technique seems to be a cost-effective and viable first-line treatment in the early stages of osteoarthritis of the great toe, there is no doubt that ultimately the successful regeneration or restoration of hyaline cartilage would provide the best long-term results in the pursuit of reestablishing a functional and pain-free joint.[1] Unfortunately, this is currently a very daunting, technically challenging, and expensive task relative to microfracture.

Several investigators have attempted to encourage the new growth of hyaline cartilage using various techniques and methods of delivery. One such technique is periosteal resurfacing, whereby an autologous periosteal flap is transferred to the cartilage defect and anchored with either a resorbable suture or fibrin glue.[82] This technique can be technically challenging and can induce donor-site morbidity. Although the original technique has been reported on for more than 15 years, it has increased in popularity more recently with the advancements in the regenerative medicine. Building on the original concept, several new techniques have recently been proposed and show great promise. First was the autologous chondrocyte implantation (ACI) or autologous chondrocyte transplantation (ACT) whereby host chondrocyte cells are injected into a cartilage defect and covered by a periosteal flap. The initial results have been quite favorable compared with microfracture techniques in that 1 year later, there was a much higher concentration of hyaline cartilage versus fibrocartilage in the ACI group.[83] Another technique that has recently been introduced and demonstrates efficacy compared with ACI is matrix-induced chondrocyte implantation (MACI), whereby host chondrocyte cells are imbedded into a collagen medium that is used as a cellular scaffold and implanted into the defect without the need for a periosteal flap or suturing, thus eliminating the need for another donor site.[84,85] Human amniotic membrane has also been suggested as a viable medium to host autologous chondrocytes, especially when seeded on the stromal side. In the initial studies in animal models, there may actually be advantages with the use of this tissue because of its unique antiscarring, antiinflammatory, and immune privilege.[86] Although most of the research for ACT and MACI has been performed either in animal models or in the knee, future applications for cartilage repair in the foot and ankle are promising.

Another method of patching osteochondral defects is with chondral transplantation techniques, such as osteochondral articular transplant (OAT). Although this technique has been described in other areas of the body, there has been very few reports involving the first MPJ, and the technique seems to be limited to focal defects whereby the surrounding cartilage is in otherwise excellent condition. Title and colleagues[87] described a protocol whereby they performed a local-shift osteochondral plug from the viable dorsal one-third portion of the metatarsal head with good success. Other autologous osteochondral donor sites for OATs have included the medial aspect of the talar head and the lateral portion of the ipsilateral lateral femoral condyle.[88] Allograft-based OATs procedures can be used in larger defects or if the donor site is not available, although true chondrocyte viability and incorporation rates versus autologous-based grafts have not been fully understood.[89]

Another promising area of recent development in cartilage regenerative techniques is the implantation of particulated articular cartilage using either the Cartilage Autograft Implantation System (DePuy/Mitek, Raynham, MA) or the DeNovo Natural Tissue (ISTO, St Louis, MO), which uses juvenile cartilage allograft tissue.[90] The main advantage of these techniques is that they are greatly simplified and require only one surgery and one operative site, significantly reducing the morbidity of multiple procedures and/or the need for a secondary donor site. Although reports in literature are limited regarding the viability of these techniques, short-term studies demonstrating both procedures to be safe, feasible, and effective, with improvements in subjective patient scores, and with MRI evidence of good defect fill in the knee.[91]

Despite continued advancement toward tissue engineering of functional articular cartilage via regenerative medicine, significant challenges still remain. Although the aforementioned procedures are focused on reestablishing the foundation of the articular surface through the encouragement of hyaline cartilage regeneration via the development and use of stem cells and various collagen-based scaffolds, one must not ignore the condition of surrounding articular environment, namely, the joint capsule and the overall health of synovial tissue. An emerging and exciting field of tribology will likely pave the way to furthering engineered cartilage therapies and will aim to incorporate approaches and methods for improved functional lubrication likely warranting a shift in the articular cartilage tissue–engineering paradigm by an increased understanding of supportive tribosupplementation, pharmacologic, and cell-based articular therapies.[92] For example, PRP and bone marrow aspirate concentrate have been proposed as important biologic adjuncts to cartilage repair techniques by the downregulation of inflammatory and catabolic processes.[93] Of course, the future of restorative medicine as it pertains to the treatment of osteoarthritic changes of the first MPJ joint is exciting and will likely be an area of extreme growth as technology advances.

JOINT-DESTRUCTIVE PROCEDURES FOR HALLUX RIGIDUS: IMPLANT ARTHROPLASTY

Although the idea of using artificial replacements of the great toe joint for the treatment of advanced hallux rigidus in not new, despite recent advancements, it has not displaced arthrodesis as the gold standard treatment (**Fig. 19**). Implant arthroplasty has been available for greater than 60 years and has undergone a great deal of maturation and change with advancing technologies and an increased appreciation of the functional biomechanics of the first MPJ. The quest to become as predictable and reliable as other joint replacements, such as the knee or hip, has been quite difficult because there is no distinct technique or design that has reigned supreme in the effort to mimic the original functional state of the joint artificially. In fact, a review of the current literature demonstrates that the overall success and benefits of implants is often intertwined with higher complication rates and the likelihood that patients with implant arthroplasty may require further revision surgery at some point.[94–96] One simply

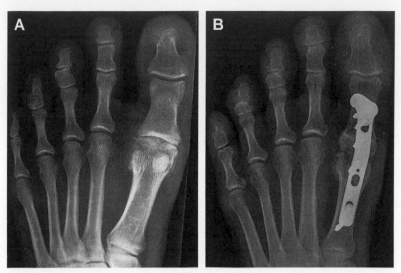

Fig. 19. (A, B) End-staged hallux limitus with pain at midrange of motion being treated with a primary arthrodesis of the first MPJ.

cannot argue against the higher success rates of a well-performed fusion, especially when it comes to addressing the pain component secondary to the advancing degenerative changes associated with the later stages of hallux rigidus.[32,94] On the other hand, arthrodesis achieves its success by means of a sacrifice of functional motion. In a perfect world where one could rely on the long-term predictability and efficacy of implant arthroplasty, the authors think that implant arthroplasty would displace arthrodesis as the gold standard treatment because of its ability to not only adequately address pain but also to avoid sacrificing motion and function. Unfortunately, implant arthroplasty remains somewhat unpredictable and is, therefore, unproven as a superior solution versus fusion for the treatment of end-stage hallux rigidus.

Perhaps the biggest challenge of implant arthroplasty is that it is almost impossible to artificially mimic the true nature of the native joint from both the anatomic and kinematic viewpoints. Engineered implants are nonorganic and, therefore, do not share the same biomechanical properties and elastic modulus of healthy hyaline cartilage over viable subchondral bone.[97,98] Also, implant arthroplasty is mechanical in nature and is, therefore, subject to breakdown over time. A marriage between metal, bone, and cartilage is also an unproven and evolving art/science. The lack of a consensus regarding proper patient candidacy, limited survivorship, increased complication rates associated with implant arthroplasty, and the limited availability of evidence-based follow-up studies have likely stifled the popularity and endorsement of implant arthroplasty in the foot and ankle surgical community. With that being said, numerous product development companies and manufacturers have continued to focus on the pursuit of creating an implant that challenges fusion as the gold standard. To achieve this, the following questions must be answered: Can a motion-sparing implant arthroplasty equal the reliability of fusion and effectiveness of pain relief and surpass it in regard to the restoration of near normal biomechanics? If not, does implant arthroplasty have a role as a viable temporary solution for patients who wish to avoid fusion or would like a more functional result than what a resectional arthroplasty could provide? There are several new promising implantation arthroplasty devices that have become available more recently that have strived to address and eliminate some of the documented risks and shortcomings of earlier generational devices. The following section attempts to summarize the current literature regarding implant arthroplasty and provide an overview of the available products/companies that provide alternatives to fusion.

IMPLANT ARTHROPLASTY AS AN ALTERNATIVE

As noted earlier, there are many surgical options available for the treatment of hallux rigidus, especially in the early stages. However, as the condition progresses toward its end stage, the need for a joint-destructive procedure becomes more relevant. The ultimate choice should depend on the severity of the disease, the desired activity level of the patients, bone quality, surgeons experience, knowledge of the risks of each alternative, and the patients' realistic expectations about the surgical intervention in both the short- and long-terms.[3,16,99] Although arthrodesis seems to be the most accepted end-stage joint-destructive procedures in the literature for younger and more active patients, several investigators advocate the use of resectional arthroplasty in older, more sedentary patients because of the reported early pain relief and less debilitative postoperative rehabilitation regimen.[68,69] On the other hand, well-educated and younger patients requiring a joint-destructive procedure, who have a more active lifestyle, may elect to avoid a dysfunctional joint and pursue implant arthroplasty.[99] The National Institute for Health and Clinical Excellence concluded that available evidence on the safety and effectiveness of artificial replacement of the first MPJ seems adequate to support the use of this procedure but acknowledges that there is limited evidence of the long-term durability of this approach.[100]

EVOLUTION AND REVOLUTION OF IMPLANT ARTHROPLASTY

Implant arthroplasty involving the great toe dates back to the early 1950s. The first reported design was derived from acrylic methacrylate anchored by bone cement in 1951 by Endler.[101] This particular implant aimed to restore the base of the proximal phalanx. Also around that same time, Townley and Taranow[96] introduced the BioPro proximal phalangeal hemiarthroplasty implant (BioPro, Port Huron, MI). The implant, which is made available in 3 evenly graded sizes, is designed to replace only the articular surface of the proximal phalanx, with minimal resection of bone stock. The follow-up at 8 months to 33 years after surgery revealed good or excellent clinical results in 95% of the patients. They concluded that the biomechanics of the hallux MPJ remained unaffected, and problems associated with prosthetic wear or mechanical failure were not encountered.[96] This particular implant paved the way for the future development of the metallic unipolar hemiarthroplasty devices. Shortly after, both Swanson and Seeburger[102,103] unsuccessfully attempted to design metatarsal head replacements, which ultimately failed secondary to the type of materials used. Implant arthroplasty did not really become popularized until the mid 1960s to early 1970s when Swanson redesigned his original implant device to include the use of silicone. The Silastic (Dow Corning Corporation, Midland, Michigan) great toe implant was comprised of a silicone cap on a single stem that was meant to act as a stabilizing spacer following the performance of a Keller resectional arthroplasty.[102,104] After disappointing early results riddled with fractures of the material, foreign-body reactions, stiffness, and permanent deformation leading to high failure rates, double-stemmed (bipolar) implants were introduced like the Laporta, Suter, and Lawrence designs.[105–107] Although they had slightly different methods of achieving dorsiflexion, these implants were designed to retain the normal function of the flexor halluces brevis and sesamoid apparatus.[106] Although the initial results were promising in regard to pain relief, longer follow-up reports revealed a high incidence in the formation of exogenous bone around the implant radiographically, painful keratotic transfer lesions to the lesser MPJ, and limited amounts of plantar flexion, with the frequency of failure being related to the duration of implant use.[14,106,108]

Because of the apparent limitations of the initial silicone implants, alternative-material (metallic, ceramic, polymer, and metal alloy) unipolar and bipolar systems have been developed.[3] Several metallic press-fit hemi and total arthroplasty devices have since been developed and have been reported to have varying degrees of success relative to other joint-destructive procedures.[14]

HEMI-IMPLANTS (UNIPOLAR)

Hemi-arthroplasty implants are 1-piece, unipolar component constructs that are designed to replace and mimic the articular surface of either the metatarsal head or the proximal phalangeal base (**Figs. 20–23**). Although insurances have been slow to authorize coverage for hemi-arthroplasty in the past because of its past tumultuous history regarding the initial failures of the early designs, more companies are starting to consider artificial joint replacement of the great toe medically necessary for persons with disabling arthritis of the first MPJ as a viable alternative to fusion. On the other hand, several companies still consider joint replacement of any method as experimental and, therefore, do not consider them for coverage.

As development moved away from Silastic hemi-arthroplasty because of the high prevalence of failure, several metal alloy-based hemi-arthroplasty designs have been developed and released.[3] Although the instrumentation and insertion method varies between manufactures, the procedure typically involves a resection and decompression of either the articular surface of the base of the proximal phalanx or head of the metatarsal, in addition to the resection and remodeling of the metatarsal head and resection of any periarticular spur formation. The prosthesis is then implanted using the specific technique associated with the particular device being used.

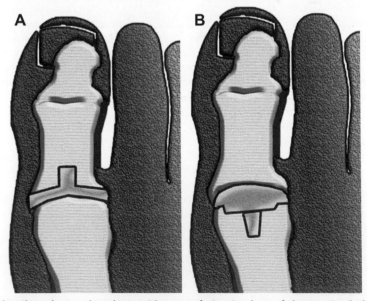

Fig. 20. (*A, B*) Implant arthroplasty with a resurfacing implant of the proximal phalangeal base and metatarsal head.

	Company	Proprietary Name	Image	Placement method	Material Type	Advancement
Phalangeal Base Resurfacing	Vilex	**Cannulated Hemi**	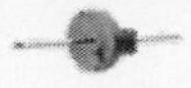	Cannulated screw fit	Titanium	Cannulated implantation
	Arthrex	**AnaToemic**	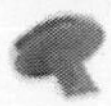	Press fit	Co-Cr-Mo	Low profile
	Biopro	**Great Toe**	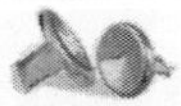	Press fit	Co-Cr-Mo	Longest follow-up studies
	Integra	**K2 Hemi Toe**	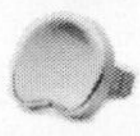	Press fit	Co-Cr-Mo	Anatomically shaped
	Metasurg	**Biomotion Cannulated**	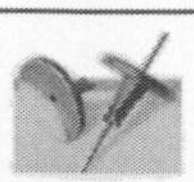	Cannulated screw fit	Titanium	Cannulated implantation
	OrthoPro	**Metal Hemi**	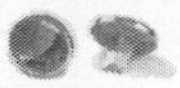	Press fit	Titanium	Dorsally elevated stem
	Osteomed	**Hemi Great Toe**	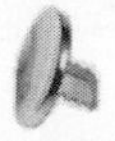	Press fit	Co-Cr-Mo	Anatomically shaped plantarly
	Tornier	**Futura Metal Hemi**	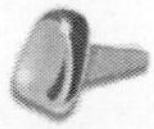	Press fit	Co-Cr-Mo	Trapezoidal shaped
	Trilliant	**3S Hemi**	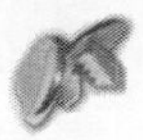	Press fit	Co-Cr-Mo	Tri-spade stem, anatomically shaped
	Wright Medical	**LPT2**	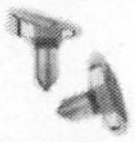	Press fit	Co-Cr-Mo	Straight and angled options
	Integra	**Movement Great toe**	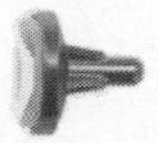	Press fit	Co-CR-Mo	Use reamer for less bone resection
	Solana	**Phalangeal Decompression Implant**	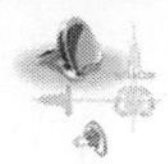	Press fit	Co-CR-Mo	Anatomic design

Fig. 21. Table representive of the current proximal phalageal base resurfacing hemi-implants. *Abbreviation:* Co-Cr-Mo, Cobalt-Chromium-Molybdenum. (Vilex: *Courtesy of* Vilex, Inc., McMinnville, TN; with permission; Arthrex: *Courtesy of* Arthrex, Inc., Naples, FL; with permission; Biopro: *Courtesy of* BioPro, Inc., Port Huron, MI; with permission; Integra: *Courtesy of* Integra, Plainsboro, NJ; with permission; Metasurg: *Courtesy of* Metasurg, Houston, TX; with permission; Orthopro: *Courtesy of* Orthopro, LLC, Salt Lake City, UT; with permission; Osteomed: *Courtesy of* OsteoMed, Addison, TX; with permission; Tornier: *Courtesy of* Tornier, Inc., Bloomington, MN; with permission; Trilliant: *Courtesy of* Trilliant Surgical, Houston, TX; with permission; Wright Medical: *Photo provided courtesy of* Wright Medical Technology, Inc; Integra: *Courtesy of* Integra, Plainsboro, NJ; with permission; Solana: *Courtesy of* Solana Surgical, Memphis, TN; with permission.)

Metatarsal Head Resurfacing					
Company	**Proprietary Name**	**Image**	**Placement method**	**Material Type**	**Advancement**
Arthrosurface	*Hemicap*	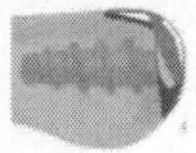	Press fit on post	Co-Cr-Mo	Dorsal phalange
Osteomed	*Encompass*	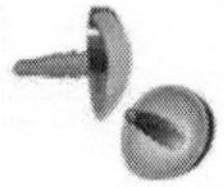	Press fit	Co-Cr-Mo, Ti	Single piece low profile stem
Solana	*Metatarsal Decompression Implant*	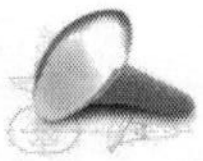	Press fit	Co-Cr-Mo	Dorsal 2/3 met-head decompression
Vilex	*Cannulated Hemi*	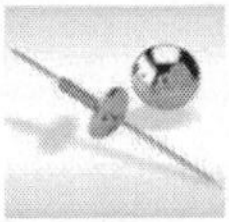	Cannulated screw fit	Titanium	Vilex
Integra	*Movement Great Toe*	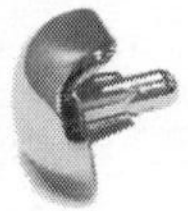	Press Fit	Co-Cr-Mo	Dorsal phalange. Surgeon also has option to resurface the base of the proximal phalanx

Fig. 22. Table is representative of the current metatarsal head resurfacing hemi-implants. *Abbreviation:* Ti, Titanium. (*Arthrosurface: Courtesy of Arthrosurface, Franklin, MA; with permission; Osteomed: Courtesy of OsteoMed, Addison, TX; with permission; Solana: Courtesy of Solana Surgical, Memphis, TN; with permission; Vilex: Courtesy of Vilex, Inc., McMinnville, TN; with permission; Integra: Courtesy of Integra, Plainsboro, NJ; with permission.*)

Company	Name	Image	Cement	Material Type	Number of components
Integra	Kinetic Great Toe	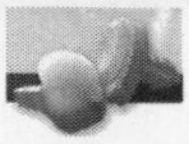	Press fit	Cr-Co-Ti, PE	2
	Movement Great Toe	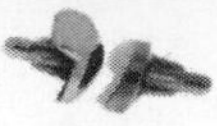	Press fit	Cr-Co-Ti, PE	2
Merete	ToeMobile	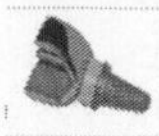	Press fit	Cr-Co-Ti, PE	2
Osteomed	Bio-Action	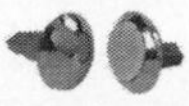	Cement	Cr-Co-Ti, PE	2
	Reflexion	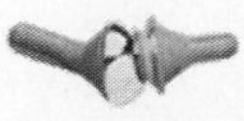	Cement	Cr-Co-Ti, PE	3
Tornier	Futura classic flexible	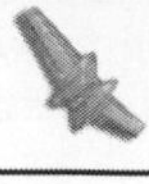	Press fit	Silicone without grommets	1
	Futura primus flexible	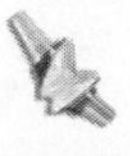	Press fit	Silicone with grommets	1
Wright Medical	Swanson Flexible	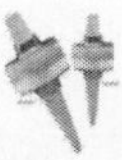	Press fit	Silicone with grommets	1

Fig. 23. Table is representative of the current total great toe joint implant device options. *Abbreviations:* Cr-Co-Ti, Cobalt-Chromium-Titanium; PE, Polyethylene. (Integra: *Courtesy of* Integra, Plainsboro, NJ; with permission; Merete: *Courtesy of* Merete Medical GmbH, Berlin, Germany; with permission; Osteomed: *Courtesy of* OsteoMed, Addison, TX; with permission; Tornier: *Courtesy of* Tornier, Inc., Bloomington, MN; with permission; Wright Medical: *Photo provided courtesy of* Wright Medical Technology, Inc.)

Current metallic-based hemi-arthroplasty has not been proven to be a superior alternative when compared with other surgical alternatives for end-staged hallux rigidus. Although some studies report that it is not as reliable as either fusion or re-sectional arthroplasty,[32,33,68,94] others demonstrate high long-term success rates.[2,3,109,110] In a most recent multicenter retrospective review, a review of the outcome for arthrodesis, hemi-implant, and resectional arthroplasty, Kim and colleagues[3] concluded that the most common complication in the hemi-implant group was exogenous heterotopic bone formation. In their study, the median total modified AOFAS score was 90 for the arthrodesis group, 80 for the hemi-implant group, and 92 for the resectional arthroplasty group. Nevertheless, they still thought that the patient satisfaction rates between the groups were relatively similar.

When reviewing the literature, one must keep in mind that there are many factors that need consideration in determining whether or not implant arthroplasty should have a significant role in the recommended treatment algorithm for end-staged hallux rigidus. Although several studies have attempted to compare the long-term outcomes of fusion versus joint replacement, they have very different goals from the onset and are, therefore, difficult to directly compare.[111] The measure of a successful fusion is usually based on pain-relief scores, radiographic and clinical evidence of fusion, and the postoperative static position of the hallux. Although there are several potential well-documented complications that can occur with this surgical approach, once the joint has successfully fused, the reliance on the hardware typically becomes obsolete and can be safely removed without sacrificing the integrity of the fusion.[15,32,99] On the other hand, the nature of joint replacement involves a high long-term reliance on the survivorship of the implant-to-bone interface; avoidance of scar tissue or bony buildup surrounding the artificial joint; and in the case of hemi-arthroplasty, the viability and health of the non-resurfaced articular surface. Although one can compare fusions based on patient satisfaction rates, tolerability, and pain scores, a functional comparison is much more difficult to assess because of the different end goals of an implant, which is to restore functional motion in addition to pain relief.[3] This topic is an evolving debate that is occurring with the ultimate treatment of end-staged arthritis of the ankle joint where, despite higher complication rates, we are now seeing patients and select surgeons favoring the pursuit of motion-sparing techniques with further advancements in implant design, materials, and implantation techniques.[112,113] The key focus of artificial implantation really should be on the true salvageability of the implant. If the implant has a relatively small imprint requiring minimal bone resection, then in the event of failure, it may be revised with a conversion to another hemi- or total arthroplasty with greater bone resection, an excisional arthroplasty with or without a biologic spacer, or more easily converted to a salvage fusion (**Fig. 24**).[15,67,88,94,114]

When determining what side of the joint to replace, the most widely accepted practice is to evaluate the extent of destruction of the articular surface of both the base of the proximal phalanx and the head of the metatarsal and replace the surface that seems to have the most damage (**Fig. 25**). Although phalangeal base implants have been more commonly used in the past, several companies have launched metatarsal head resurfacing implants in light of more recent observations in the literature that suggest the metatarsal head is usually more damaged and, therefore, should be the focus of resurfacing implantation.[115] Currently, literature is lacking in comparison of outcomes between the 2 types of resurfacing implants. In the authors' personal experience and use of 3 different metatarsal head implant designs, although they tend to

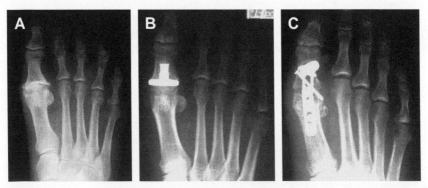

Fig. 24. (*A, B*) Preoperative and postoperative radiographs of a hemi-arthroplasty resurfacing implant. Although the patient had improved range of motion and decreased pain at 6 months, there was still residual pain with maximal dorsiflexion in the dorsal-lateral aspect of the joint. (*C*) The patient elected to have the implant removed and converted to fusion. Intraoperatively, there seemed to be hypertrophic capsular tissue interposed between the implant and the metatarsal head consistent with the area of residual pain. This procedure was performed with the use of conical reamers and without the need of an interpositional bone graft because of the limited amount of bone resected with the initial surgery.

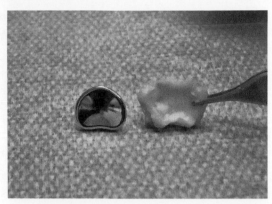

Fig. 25. Demonstration of significantly degenerated articular cartilage of the proximal phalangeal base. In this case, a decision was made to resurface the base with an anatomic-shaped metallic hemi-arthroplasty.

rival the proximal phalangeal hemi-arthroplasty devices in regard to pain relief, they also seem to be associated with a greater degree of postoperative stiffness and a reduction of functional motion (**Fig. 26**). Further studies are warranted to evaluate the long-term efficacy of hemi-implantation of the metatarsal head versus the base

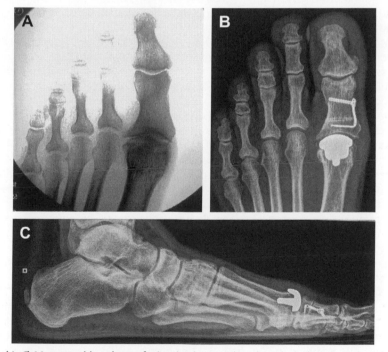

Fig. 26. (A–C) Metatarsal head resurfacing implant with a dorsal phalange. A dorsal-closing wedge osteotomy was performed in an attempt to further decompress the joint and improve the postoperative range of motion. Although the patient had much better range of motion of the toe at 6 months postoperatively than before the surgery, the motion was significantly reduced compared with his unaffected foot. The patient claimed that he experienced 95% improvement in his original pain following the procedure.

of the proximal phalanx. Some of the more commonly used hemi-implants are briefly discussed here along with a brief description of their unique design features.

PHALANGEAL-BASE RESURFACING HEMI-ARTHROPLASTY DEVICES

- *AnaToemic Phalangeal Hemiprosthesis* (Arthrex, Naples, FL): The AnaToemic resurfaces the proximal phalanx and promotes a 2.4-mm head. According to the manufacturer, this size of head requires minimal resection of the base of the proximal phalanx, allowing patients to maintain the flexor attachment. It is comprised of cobalt-chrome and uses a pilot punch to accurately place the implant.
- *BioPro GREAT TOE* (BioPro, Port Huron, MI): The BioPro is a hemi-implant that resurfaces the proximal phalangeal base and has been around since its introduction in 1952. It is available in a porous and a nonporous cobalt chrome. It is indicated to replace the base of the proximal phalanx and has a diamond-shaped stem providing intramedullary fixation.
- *The Integra K2 Hemi Toe Implant System* (Integra, Plainsboro, NJ): The K2 Hemi is made of cobalt chrome with a titanium plasma-coated stem. It is designed for the proximal phalanx; on the inferior aspect of the implant base, there is a slight groove for the flexor hallucis longus tendon. It also features a suture hole allowing the flexor hallucis brevis (FHB) to be sutured to the implant to add flexion power to the proximal phalanx. There is a cutting guide that allows you to take the exact amount of bone needed to place the implant, which measurers 2 mm in width.
- *BioMotion First MPJ Cannulated Hemi System* (Metasurg, Houston, TX): The BioMotion is designed for the proximal phalanx that offers the minimal bone resection that is needed to maintain the flexor tendon attachment sites. It is a cannulated implant, allowing precise alignment. It has a tapered stem and offers 5 color-coded sizes.
- *The Metal Hemi* (OrthroPro, Salt Lake City, UT): The Metal Hemi is a titanium implant used to replace the base of the proximal phalanx. According to the manufacturer, the implant stem is dorsally elevated to allow for better, more accurate positioning and has a plantar fin to prevent rotation.
- *Futura Metal Hemi Toe (MHT)* (Tornier, Bloomington, MN): The MHT features a cobalt chrome, single-stemmed resurfacing prosthesis for the base of the proximal phalanx that has a titanium plasma coating along the intramedullary stem to promote osseous integration. It has a trapezoidal articular surface to be congruent with the metatarsal head and is rounded dorsally to decrease impingement on the metatarsal head. It has a thinned inferior surface to preserve the flexor hallucis brevis attachment site. The stem is trapezoidal and angled to protect the plantar cortex.

There was a follow-up study that evaluated patients with a Futura MHT implant for an average of 96 months postoperatively. There were 13 implants evaluated (11 patients total), and they found all MPJs stable and well aligned clinically. There were lucencies noted at the base of the implants but not around the stem in 11 implants. The first MPJ range of motion averaged 17° of plantar flexion with 47° of dorsiflexion and averaged a total of 64° of total range of motion. More than half of the patients had a recurrence of the dorsal osteophyte, and 3 patients noticed a decreased amount of dorsiflexion. Koenig scores averaged 80, with AOFAS forefoot scores averaging 83. Ten of the 11 patients were satisfied with the results of the implant.[109,116]

- *3S Hemi Implant* (Trilliant Surgical, Houston, TX): The 3S Hemi Implant was designed to resurface the base of the proximal phalanx. Its design features a tris-pade stem for maximum contact between the implant and bone and promotes a anatomic concaved shape. It is made of cobalt chromium and has a color coded instrumentation kit.
- *Cannulated Hemi Implant (CHI) System* (Vilex, McMinnville, TN): The CHI system has 2 different options to choose from based on the deterioration of the articular cartilage of the joint. Vilex CHI has hemi-implants available in elliptical and concave shapes to replace the base of the proximal phalanx. There are also spherical and convex shapes to replace the metatarsal to resurface the meta-tarsal head. All the implants are cannulated to allow for precise positioning within the joint. There are also 2 positioning holes to allow for suturing the implant to the soft tissue, if the surgeon desires to.
- *LPT2 Great Toe Implant* (Wright Medical, Arlington, TN): The LPT2 implant is a titanium implant that resurfaces the base of the proximal phalanx and uniquely comes in straight or angled designs. The angled implant can correct or accom-modate an increased PASA on the metatarsal head. The implant also has man-ufactured suture holds if needed. If using the angled implant to address and increase the PASA, it is important to place the wider portion laterally.
- *Swanson Titanium Great Toe Implant* (Wright Medical, Arlington, TN): The Swan-son Titanium Great Toe is an intramedullary stemmed implant that replaces the proximal third of the proximal phalanx. The implant is made to preserve joint space by being surrounded by a fibrous supporting capsule. It is available in 5 sizes.

    In a study of 10 patients (13 implants), followed up on an average of 66 months, pain was absent in 6 toes and mild and occasional in 5 toes. In 12 of the 13 implants, there was no limitation of activity, and the patient with limited activity resolved the issue by wearing extradepth shoes. At 5.5 years follow-up, 86% of patients were satisfied. The average Koenig score was 88 and the average AOFAS forefoot score was 86. All patients were satisfied, but it was noted that all 10 patients had subsidence and lucency around the implant.[117]
- *Hemi Great Toe Implant* (OsteoMed, Addison, TX): The Osteomed Hemi Great Toe Implant is a one piece implant that resurfaces the base of the proximal pha-lanx of the first metatarsal phalangeal joint. According to the manufacturer, it is an anatomic-based design that focuses on alignment to allow for improved and pain-free range of motion. The Hemi instrument tray includes trials, sizers, punch and impactor for convenient placement of the device. It is available in four implant sizes and is low profile resulting in minimal bone resection during implantation.[118]

METATARSAL HEAD RESURFACING HEMI-ARTHROPLASTY DEVICES

- *Arthrosurface HemiCAP DF Toe Resurfacing System* (Arthrosurface, Franklin, MA): The Arthrosurface HemiCAP is indicated for the first metatarsal head resur-facing. It is a 2-piece, single-component implant with a cancellous taper post and 2 designs (with and without a dorsal phalange) for an articular resurfacing cap. According to the manufacturer, it is designed to provide stable and immobile implant fixation and is made of cobalt chromium alloy with a titanium surface coating and a titanium alloy taper post. The metatarsal head can be decom-pressed before the insertion of the implant with the included metatarsal head reamers.

- *Metatarsal Decompression Implant System (MDI)* (Solana Surgical, Memphis, TN): The MDI is a metatarsal head resurfacing implant. It is made of titanium featuring a cobalt chromium coating. There are 4 available sizes, and it can provide up to 3 mm of decompression of the metatarsal. The implant is oval shaped, with a toroidal articular surface of the head to distribute gait forces. According to the manufacturer, it primarily resurfaces the upper two-thirds of the metatarsal head in an attempt to prevent scaring and capsular adhesions from the plantar capsular tissue. The proximal stem is tapered and rectangular distally to prevent rotation.
- *CHI System* (Vilex, McMinnville, TN): See the description in the previous section.
- *The EnCompass Metatarsal Resurfacing Implant* (OsteoMed, Addison, TX): The EnCompass Metatarsal Resurfacing Implant is designed to replace the metatarsal head. It has a concave spherical surface that is coated with titanium plasma and hydroxyapatite. It has several sizes, is one piece, and has a proximal stem that is fixated into the metatarsal canal. It has a 4-finned stem to provide stability and prevent rotation.
- *Integra MOVEMENT Great Toe System* (Integra, Plainsboro, NJ): See the discussion later regarding total joint arthroplasty.

TOTAL MTP JOINT REPLACEMENT (BIPOLAR)

Several attempts have been made to design total metatarsal joint replacements since first being introduced more than 50 years ago; but to date, none have reached wide acceptance. Although total joint replacement remains the ultimate reliable solution for both knee and hip osteoarthritis and may be a viable option in ankle osteoarthritis, artificial replacement of the first MPJ has not been established as a standard of care for osteoarthritis of the great toe.[14] Despite its initial success in relieving symptoms, the first- and second-generational joint replacements with a flexible, hinged silicone were abandoned because of poor durability and a rather high failure rate.[106] The third-generation Silastic implants were redesigned for insertion with titanium grommets to reduce the stress applied to the implant-to-bone interface in an attempt to increase the survival of the arthroplasty.[12]

Some insurance companies consider total prosthetic replacement arthroplasty with Silastic implants medically necessary for persons with disabling arthritis of the first MPJ and that it is a viable alternative to fusion. On the other hand, several insurance companies do not provide coverage for replacement arthroplasty using total metallic implants, stating that they are experimental and investigational for the treatment of hallux rigidus, degenerative arthritis, and other indications involving the MPJ because their effectiveness has not been established in. A systematic review of the literature by Brewster[119] revealed that despite good results in both groups, arthrodesis achieves better functional outcomes than total joint replacement. The median postoperative AOFAS score for joint replacement was 83 out of 100 (ranging from 74–95) and 82 out of 100 (ranging from 78–89) for arthrodesis in the same study. The median revision rate in joint replacements was 7% and 0% for arthrodesis. What remains clear is that total replacement of the first MPJ has come a long way since its inception and is a challenging and yet promising field of forefoot reconstructive surgery. Further research on the implant design seems to be mandatory to overcome the problems that lead to the need for revision.[120–122] A brief description of the currently available first MPJ implants approved by the Food and Drug Administration are discussed later.

- *Integra MOVEMENT Great Toe System* (Integra, Plainsboro, NJ): The Movement Great Toe System allows the surgeon to determine intraoperatively the extent of the cartilage wear and to decide whether or not a hemi-arthroplasty versus a total-arthroplasty is more appropriate. The implants have a cobalt chrome artic- ular surface, with titanium plasma spray promoting osseous integration. It has a cylindrical 4-fin stem for stability. The metatarsal implant specifically features a dorsal flange to help prevent formation of osteophytes. The proximal phalanx implant is reamed into place to avoid the disturbance of the flexor halluces brevis insertion while minimizing bone resection. It also has suture holes for flexor reat- tachment if the flexor apparatus is compromised.

- *The Integra Kinetik Great Toe Implant System* (Integra, Plainsboro, NJ): The Kinetik Great Toe is a 2-piece, nonconstrained implant for the total replacement of the first MPJ. This 2-component system offers interchangeable components and a dorsal flange on a metatarsal component that extends the dorsal range of motion. This particular implant is used less often because of the more popular MOVEMENT, which was recently acquired from Ascension orthopedics.

- *ToeMobile Anatomic Great Toe Resurfacing System* (Merete Medical, New Windsor, NY): The ToeMobile is a 2-piece nonconstrained prosthesis that re- places the MPJ by complete functional preservation of the joint while maintaining the sesamoid complex. The prosthesis consists of an anatomically shaped and polished metatarsal implant made of Cobalt-Chromium-Molybdenum (CoCrMo), which glides on a polyethylene inlay that is preassembled on a conically shaped phalangeal component made of titanium alloy Ti-6Al-4V.

- *The OsteoMed Bio-Action Toe Great Toe Implant* (OsteoMed, Addison, TX): The Bio-Action Toe is no longer available on the market. See the OsteoMed ReFlexion first MPJ Implant System. A study reviewed 36 Bio-Action Great Toe Implants (in 32 patients) at an average of 47 months. There was noted to be significant improvement in dorsiflexion and first MTPJ range of motion. Twenty-eight patients had an improvement in function. Only 3 patients continued to have pain. There was subsidence of the implant 12 (33%), but patients did not report a change in satisfaction. Twenty-eight patients reported excellent or good satisfaction with the implant, with only 3 rating it poor.[118]

- *The Osteomed ReFlexion 1st MPJ Implant System* (OsteoMed, Addison, TX): This device is a 3-piece nonconstrained implant system for the primary and revision reconstruction of the first MPJ with a cone-in-cone implant design. It has re- placed the Bio-Action Great Toe Implant in OsteoMed's portfolio. All compo- nents are interchangeable and available in 3 sizes. The 17° orientation of the metatarsal component accommodates the angle of declination of the metatarsal head. In their prospective study with a 39-month follow-up, Fuhrmann and col- leagues[120] revealed encouraging results for pain relief and follow-up using the Reflexion endoprosthesis on 41 patients (43 joints). The AOFAS score improved from 51 points preoperatively to 74 points postoperatively.

- *The Futura Primus Flexible Great Toe (model FGT)* (Tornier, Bloomington, MN): The Futura Primus implant is a third-generation Silastic prosthesis designed to supplement first MPJ arthroplasty. The implant is constructed from ULTRASIL (Evonik Industries, Wesseling, Germany) medical-grade silicone elastomer and includes titanium grommets. The inferior aspect of the distal hinge buttress is angled to minimize interference with the flexor hallucis brevis attachment site and the sesamoid apparatus.

- *The Futura Classic Flexible Great Toe* (Tornier, Bloomington, MN): The Futura Flexible Great Toe implant is also a third-generation prosthesis designed to supplement first MPJ arthroplasty. Constructed from ULTRASIL medical-grade silicone elastomer, the Classic offers Futura's patented axial offset hinge and

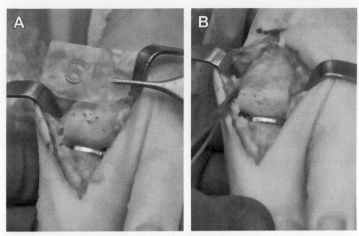

Fig. 27. (A, B) A hybrid technique with a metatarsal cheilectomy, microfracture of the metatarsal head, hemi-arthroplasty of the proximal phalangeal base, and use an orthobiologic amniotic membrane barrier used to cover the exposed metatarsal bone and prevent capsular scarring and adhesions postoperatively.

other advanced design features while maintaining the surgical technique of the previous generation's joint replacements.

SUMMARY

Surgical options for end-staged hallux rigidus are increasing at a dizzying rate. Although fusion remains the gold standard treatment based on its long-term predictability, there are many emerging technologies that may one day surpass fusion as the go-to option. Currently, the foot and ankle space is the fastest growing segment of orthopedics manufacturing. With the greater emphasis in research and development of new foot and ankle products, we are bound to see some truly innovative solutions come to the market in the near future. The recent expansion into orthobiologics will likely serve as the foundation that will catapult us into the future with the exciting world of regenerative medicine, where ultimately, the need for joint-destructive procedures could become a thing of the past (**Fig. 27**).

In regard to where we stand now, there are several viable treatment alternatives to fusion for end-staged hallux rigidus. Each treatment must not only be tailored to fit the needs and expectations of the patient but also fall within the surgeon's comfort level, type of training, and practice philosophy. When selecting a fusion alternative technique, patients must be fully informed and comfortable with the potential pitfalls or complications typically associated with it. Perhaps more focus should be aimed at delaying or preventing the need for fusion in our treatment pathways. If implant arthroplasty is chosen, whether it is an artificial joint or a biologic spacer, the surgeon must also assess the salvageability of that particular technique or device. Also, greater follow-up studies need to be performed to gain a better understanding of the newer-generational devices and treatment methodologies. Either way, as with other major joints of the body, focus should always be on pushing the envelope to recreate or restore the joint to its disease-free state. Although there is no clear consensus regarding what is the best treatment pathway for end-staged hallux rigidus, the one thing that is certain is that the options in each of our personal algorithms will continue to expand and change based on the updated literature and our own practice experiences. Ultimately, the real gold standard technique should be one that reliably restores normal foot function, eliminates pain, achieves good alignment and cosmesis, and significantly improves the patients' quality of life both immediately and long term, while preserving future treatment options should the original plan fail.

REFERENCES

1. Gali M, Hyer C. Hallux rigidus: what lies beyond fusion, resections arthroplasty, and implants. Clin Podiatr Med Surg 2011;28(2):385–403.
2. Giza E, Sullivan M, Ocel D, et al. First metatarsophalangeal hemiarthroplasty for hallux rigidus. Int Orthop 2010;34:1193–8.
3. Kim PJ, Hatch D, DiDomenico LA, et al. A multicenter retrospective review of outcomes for arthrodesis, hemi-metallic joint implant, and resectional arthroplasty in the surgical treatment of end-stage hallux rigidus. J Foot Ankle Surg 2012;51:50–6.
4. Wulker N. Hallux Rigidus. Turk J Arthroscopic Surg 2000;11(1):95–103.
5. Cotterill JM. Condition of stiff great toe in adolescents. Edinb Med J 1877;33:459–62.
6. Muscarella VJ, Hetherington VG. Hallux limitus and hallux rigidus. In: Hetherington VJ, editor. Hallux valgus and forefoot surgery. New York: Churchill Livingstone; 1994. p. 313–25.
7. DuVries HL. Surgery of the foot. St Louis (MO): Mosby; 1959.
8. Nilsonne H. Hallux rigidus and its treatment. Acta Orthop Scand 1930;1:295–302.
9. Zammet GV, Menz HB, Munteanu SE, et al. Interventions for treating osteoarthritis of the big toe joint. Cochrane Database Syst Rev 2010;(9):CD007809. p. 1–21.
10. Nawiczenski DA, Baumhauer JF, Umberger BR. Relationship between clinical measurements and motion of the first metatarsophalangeal joint during gait. J Bone Joint Surg Am 1999;81:370–6.
11. Van Saase JL, Can Romunde LK, Cats A. Epidemiology of osteoarthritis: Zoetermeer survey. Comparison of osteoarthritis in a Dutch population with that in 10 other populations. Ann Rheum Dis 1989;48:271–80.
12. Yee G, Lau J. Current concepts review: hallux rigidus. Foot Ankle Int 2008;29(6):637–46.
13. Coughlin MJ, Shurnas PS. Hallux rigidus: demographics, etiology, and radiographic assessment. Foot Ankle Int 2003;24(10):731–43.
14. DeCarbo WT, Lupica J, Hyer C. Modern techniques in hallux rigidus surgery. Clin Podiatr Med Surg 2011;28:361–83.
15. Deland JT, Williams BR. Surgical management of hallux rigidus. J Am Acad Orthop Surg 2012;20:347–58.
16. Keiserman LS, Sammarco VJ, Sammarco GJ. Surgical treatment of hallux rigidus. Foot Ankle Clin 2005;10(1):75–96.
17. Easley ME, Davis WH, Anderson RB. Intermediate to long-term follow-up of medial-approach dorsal cheilectomy for hallux rigidus. Foot Ankle Int 1999;20(3):147–52.
18. Beeson P, Phillips C, Corr S, et al. Classification systems for hallux rigidus; a review of the literature. Foot Ankle Int 2008;29(4):407–14.
19. Jorge L, Feres C, Teles VE. Topical preparations for pain relief: efficacy and patient adherence. J Pain Res 2011;4:11–24.
20. Grady JF, Axe TM, Zager EJ, et al. A retrospective analysis of 772 patients with hallux limitus. J Am Podiatr Med Assoc 2002;92(2):102–8.

21. Papacrhistou G, Anagnostou S, Katsorhis T. The effect of intraarticular hydrocortisone injection on the articular cartilage of rabbits. Acta Orthop Scand Suppl 1997;275:132–4.

22. Piper SL, Kramer JD, Kim HT, et al. Effects of local anesthetics on articular cartilage. Am J Sports Med 2011;39(10):2245–53.

23. Pons M, Alvarez F, Solana J, et al. Sodium hyaluronate in the treatment of hallux rigidus: a single-blinded, randomized study. Foot Ankle Int 2007;28(1): 38–42.

24. Shoor S. Review: viscosupplementation for knee osteoarthritis reduces pain and improves function. Evid Based Med 2011;11(1):12.

25. Gonzalez-Fuentes AM, Green DM, Rossen RD, et al. Intra-articular hyaluronic acid increases cartilage breakdown biomarker in patients with knee osteoarthritis. Clin Rheumatol 2010;29(6):619–24.

26. Kon E, Mandelbaum B, Buda R. Platelet-rich plasma intra-articular injection versus hyaluronic acid viscosupplementation as treatments for cartilage pathology: from early degeneration to osteoarthritis. Arthroscopy 2011;27(11):1490–501.

27. Smyth NA, Fansa AM, Murawski CD, et al. Platelet-rich plasma as a biological adjunct to the surgical treatment of osteochondral lesions of the talus. Tech Foot Ankle Surg 2012;11:18–25.

28. Akeda K, An HS, Okuma M, et al. Platelet-rich plasma stimulates porcine articular chondrocyte and matrix biosynthesis. Osteoarthritis Cartilage 2006;14:1272–80.

29. Mishra A, Tummala P, King A, et al. Buffered platelet-rich plasma enhances mesenchymal stem cell proliferation and chondrogenic differentiation. Tissue Eng Part C Methods 2009;15:431–5.

30. Kolambkar YM, Peister A, Soker S, et al. Chondrogenic differentiation of amniotic fluid-derived stem cells. J Mol Histol 2007;38(5):405–13.

31. Mackay DC, Blyth M, Rymaszewski LA. The role of cheilectomy in the treatment of hallux rigidus. J Foot Ankle Surg 1997;36(5):337–40.

32. Coughlin MJ, Shurnas PS. Hallux rigidus: grading and long term results of operative treatment. J Bone Joint Surg Am 2003;85(11):2072–88.

33. Chang TJ. Stepwise approach to hallux limitus. A surgical perspective. Clin Podiatr Med Surg 1996;13(3):449–59.

34. Waizy H, Czardybon MA, Stukenborg-Colsman C, et al. Mid- and long-term results of the joint preserving therapy of hallux rigidus. Arch Orthop Trauma Surg 2010;130(2):165–70.

35. Banks AS, McGlamry ED. Hallux limitus and rigidus. In: Banks AS, Downey MS, McGlamry ED, et al, editors. Comprehensive textbook of foot surgery. Baltimore (MD): Williams and Wilkins; 1992. p. 600–16.

36. Cochrane WA. An operation for hallux rigidus. Br Med J 1927;1:1095–6.

37. Lin J, Murphy GA. Treatment of hallux rigidus with cheilectomy using a dorsolateral approach. Foot Ankle Int 2009;30:115–9.

38. Watermann H. Die arthritis deformans grosszehengrundgelenkes. Ztschr Orthop Chir 1927;48:346–55.

39. Cavalo DJ, Cavallaro DC, Arringto LE. Ther Watermann osteotomy for hallux limitus. J Am Podiatry Assoc 1979;69(1):52–7.

40. Beeson P. The surgical treatment of hallux limitus/rigidus: a critical of the literature. Foot 2009;14(1):6–22.

41. Camasta CA, Chang TJ. Hallux limitus and Hallux rigidus. In: Banks AS, Downey MS, McGlamry ED, et al, editors. McGlamry's comprehensive textbook of foot and ankle surgery. 3rd edition. Philadelphia: Lippincott Williams & Wilkins; 2001. p. 679–710.

42. Laakman G, Green R, Green DR. The modified Watermann procedure a preliminary retrospective study. In: Camasta CA, editor. Reconstructive surgery of the foot and leg update. Tucker (GA): The Podiatry Institute; 1995. p. 128–35.
43. Feldman KA. The Green-Watermann procedure: geometric analysis and preoper-. J Foot Surg 1992;31(2):182–5.
44. Dickerson JB, Green R, Green DR. Long-term follow-up of the Green-Watermann. J Am Podiatr Med Assoc 2002;92(10):543–54.
45. Youngswick FD. Modifications of the Austin bunionectomy for treatment of metatarsus primus elevatus associated with hallux limitus. J Foot Surg 1982;21(2):114–6.
46. Radovic P, Yadav-Shah E, Choe K. Modified Youngswick procedure for hallux limitus. J Am Podiatr Med Assoc 2007;97(5):420–3.
47. Gerbert J, Moadab A, Rupley KF. Youngswick-Austin procedure: the effect of plantar arm orientation on meta-tarsal head displacement. J Foot Ankle Surg 2001;40:8.
48. Kessel L, Bonney G. Hallux rigidus in the adolescent. J Bone Joint Surg Br 1958;40(4):668–73.
49. Purvis CG, Brown JH, Kaplan EG, et al. Combination Bonney-Kessell and modified Akin procedure for hallux limitus associated with hallux abductus. J Am Podiatr Med Assoc 1977;67:236–40.
50. Kilmartin TE. Phalangeal osteotomy versus first metatarsal decompression osteotomy for the surgical treatment of hallux rigidus: a prospective study of age- matched and condition-matched patients. J Foot Ankle Surg 2005;44(1):2–12.
51. Bonney G, Macnab I. Hallux valgus and hallux rigidus: a critical survey of operative results. J Bone Joint Surg Br 1952;34(3):366–85.
52. Ronconi P, Monachino P, Baleanu PM, et al. Distal oblique osteotomy of the first metatarsal for the correction of hallux limitus and rigidus deformity. J Foot Ankle Surg 2000;39(3):154–60.
53. LaMar L, Deroy AR, Sinnot MT. Mechanical comparison of the Youngswick, sagittal V, and modified Weil osteotomies for hallux rigidus in a sawbone model. J Foot Ankle Surg 2006;45(2):70–5.
54. Drago JJ, Oloff L, Jacobs AM. A comprehensive review of hallux limitus. J Foot Surg 1984;23(3):213–20.
55. McGlamry ED, Banks AS. McGlamry's comprehensive textbook of foot and ankle surgery. 3rd edition. Chicago (IL): Lippincott Williams & Wilkins; 2001.
56. Viegas GV. Reconstruction of hallux limitus deformity using a first metatarsal sagittal-Z osteotomy. J Foot Ankle Surg 1998;37(3):204–11.
57. Blitz NM. The versatility of the Lapidus arthrodesis. Clin Podiatr Med Surg 2009;26(3):427–41.
58. Robinson SC, Frank RP. Long arm decompression osteotomy for hallux limitus. Clin Podiatr Med Surg 2005;22(2):301–7.
59. Moberg E. A simple operation for hallux rigidus. Clin Orthop Relat Res 1979;55–6.
60. Aldegheri R, Trivella G, Saleh M. Articulated distraction of the hip: conservative surgery for arthritis in young patients. Clin Orthop Relat Res 1994;301:94–101.
61. Kluesner AJ, Wukich DK. Ankle arthrodiastasis. Clin Podiatr Med Surg 2009;26(2):227–44.
62. Zgonis T, Stapleton JJ, Roukis TS. Use of circular external fixation for combined subtalar joint arthrodesis and ankle distraction. Clin Podiatr Med Surg 2008;25:745–53.

63. Talarico LM, Vito GR, Goldstein L, et al. Management of hallux limitus with distraction of the first metatarsophalangeal joint. J Am Podiatr Med Assoc 2005;95(2):121–9.
64. Abraham JS, Hassani H, Lamm BM. Hinged external fixation distraction for treatment of first metatarsophalangeal joint arthritis. J Foot Ankle Surg 2012; 51(5):604–12.
65. Hamilton WG, O'Malley MJ, Thompson FM, et al. Capsular interposition arthroplasty for severe hallux rigidus. Foot Ankle Int 1997;18:68–70.
66. Lau JT, Daniels TR. Outcomes following cheilectomy and interpositional arthroplasty in hallux rigidus. Foot Ankle Int 2001;22:462–70.
67. Mroczek KJ, Miller SD. The modified oblique Keller procedure: a technique for dorsal approach interposition arthroplasty sparing the flexor tendons. Foot Ankle Int 2003;24:521–2.
68. Kennedy JG, Chow FY, Dines J, et al. Outcomes after interpositional arthroplasty for the treatment of hallux rigidus. Clin Orthop Relat Res 2006;445:210–5.
69. Mackey RB, Thomson AB, Kwon O, et al. The modified oblique Keller capsular interpositional arthroplasty for hallux rigidus. J Bone Joint Surg Am 2010;92(10): 1938–46.
70. Roukis TS, Landsman AS, Ringstrom JB, et al. Distally based capsule-periosteum interpositional arthroplasty for hallux rigidus: indications, operative technique, and short term follow-up. J Am Podiatr Med Assoc 2003;93(5):349–66.
71. Coughlin MJ, Shurnas PJ. Soft-tissue arthroplasty for hallux rigidus. Foot Ankle Int 2003;24(9):661–72.
72. Givissis P, Symeonidis P, Christodoulou A, et al. Interposition arthroplasty of the first metatarsophalangeal joint with fascia lata allograft. J Am Podiatr Med Assoc 2008;93(5):349–66.
73. Berlet GC, Hyer CF, Lee TH, et al. Interpositional arthroplasty of the first MTP using a regenerative tissue matrix for the treatment of advanced hallux rigidus. Foot Ankle Int 2008;29(1):10–21.
74. Heller E, Robinson D. Gelfoam first metatarsophalangeal replacement/interposition arthroplasty - a case series with functional outcomes. Foot 2011;21: 119–23.
75. Blevins FT, Steadman JR, Rodrigo JJ, et al. Treatment of articular cartilage defects in athletes: an analysis of functional outcome and lesion appearance. Orthopedics 1998;21:761–7.
76. Frisbie DD, Oxford JT, Southwood L, et al. Early events in cartilage repair after subchondral bone microfracture. Clin Orthop Relat Res 2003;(407):215–27.
77. Mithoefer K, McAdams T, Williams RJ. Clinical efficacy of the microfracture technique for articular cartilage repair in the knee: an evidence-based systematic analysis. Am J Sports Med 2009;37(10):2053–63.
78. Lim HC, Bae JH, Song SH, et al. Current treatments of isolated articular cartilage lesions of the knee achieve similar outcomes. Clin Orthop Relat Res 2012; 470(8):2261–7.
79. Mithoefer K, Williams RJ 3rd, Warren RF, et al. The microfracture technique for the treatment of articular cartilage lesions in the knee. A prospective cohort study. J Bone Joint Surg Am 2005;87(9):1911–20.
80. Bojanić I, Smoljanović T, Kubat O. Osteochondritis dissecans of the first metatarsophalangeal joint: arthroscopy and microfracture technique. J Foot Ankle Surg 2011;50(5):623–5.
81. Denbath UK, Hemmady MV, Hariharan K. Indications for and technique of first metatarsal joint arthroscopy. Foot Ankle Int 2006;27(12):1049–54.

82. Zeifang F, Oberle D, Nierhoff C, et al. Autologous chondrocyte implantation using the original periosteum-cover technique versus matrix-associated autologous chondrocyte implantation: a randomized clinical trial. Am J Sports Med 2011;38(5):924–33.

83. Saris D, Vanlauwe J, Victor J, et al. Characterized chondrocyte implantation results in better structural repair when treating symptomatic cartilage defects of the knee in a randomized controlled trial versus microfracture. Am J Sports Med 2008;36(2):235–46.

84. Marlovits S, Striessnig G, Kutscha-Lissberg F, et al. Early postoperative adherence of matrix-induced autologous chondrocyte implantation for the treatment of full-thickness cartilage defects of the femoral condyle. Knee Surg Sports Traumatol Arthrosc 2005;13(6):451–7.

85. Brittberg M. Cell carriers as the next generation of cell therapy for cartilage repair: a review of the matrix-induced autologous chondrocyte implantation procedure. Am J Sports Med 2010;38(6):1259–71.

86. Chend ZJ, Park SR, Choi BH, et al. Human amniotic membrane as a delivery matrix. Tissue Eng 2007;13(4):693–702.

87. Title CI, Zaret D, Means KR Jr, et al. First metatarsal head OATS technique: an approach to cartilage damage. Foot Ankle Int 2006;27(11):1000–2.

88. Hopson M, Stone P, Paden M. First metatarsal head osteoarticular transfer system for salvage of a failed hemicap-implant: a case report. J Foot Ankle Surg 2009;48(4):483–7.

89. Fitzpatrick K, Tokish JM. Allograft OATS: decision-making and operative steps. J Knee Surg 2011;24(2):101–8.

90. Hatic SO 2nd, Berlet GC. Particulated juvenile articular cartilage graft (DeNovo NT graft) for treatment of osteochondral lesions of the talus. Foot Ankle Spec 2010;3(6):361–4.

91. Farr J, Cole BJ, Sherman S, et al. Particulated articular cartilage: CAIS and DeNovo NT. J Knee Surg 2012;25(1):23–9.

92. McNary SM, Athanasiou KA, Reddi AH. Engineering lubrication in articular cartilage. Tissue Eng Part B Rev 2012;18(2):88–100.

93. Smyth NA, Murawski CD, Haleem AM, et al. Establishing proof of concept: platelet-rich plasma and bone marrow aspirate concentrate may improve cartilage repair following surgical treatment for osteochondral lesions of the talus. World J Orthop 2012;3(7):101–8.

94. Raikin SM, Ahmad JA, Pour AE, et al. Comparison of arthrodesis and metallic hemiarthroplasty of the hallux metatarsophalangeal joint. J Bone Joint Surg Am 2007;89:1979–85.

95. Taranow WS, Moutsatson MJ, Cooper JM. Contemporary approaches to stage II and III hallux rigidus: the role of metallic hemiarthroplasty of the proximal phalanx. Foot Ankle Int 2005;10:713–28.

96. Townley CO, Taranow WS. A metallic hemiarthroplasty resurfacing prosthesis for the hallux metatarsophalangeal joint. Foot Ankle Int 1994;15:575–80.

97. Hild GA, McKee PJ. Evaluation and biomechanics of the first ray in the patient with limited motion. Clin Podiatr Med Surg 2011;28(2):245–67.

98. Botek G, Anderson MA. Etiology, pathophysiology, and staging of hallux rigidus. Clin Podiatr Med Surg 2011;28(2):229–43.

99. Brage ME, Ball ST. Surgical options for salvage of end-stage hallux rigidus. Foot Ankle Clin 2002;7(1):49–73.

100. Dillon A. Metatarsal phalangeal joint replacement of the hallux. Interventional procedures consultation document. http://www.nice.org.uk/page.aspx?o=258868.

[Online] November 2005. Available at: http://www.nice.org.uk/nicemedia/live/11188/31443/31443.pdf. Accessed September 21, 2012.

101. Endler F. Development of a prosthetic arthroplasty of the head of the first metatarsal bone, with a review of present indications. Z Orthop Grenzgeb 1951; 80(3):480–7.

102. Swanson AB. Implant arthroplasty for the great toe. Clin Orthop Relat Res 1972; 85:75–81.

103. Seeburger RH. Surgical implants of alloyed metal in joints of the feet. J Am Podiatry Assoc 1964;54:391.

104. Swanson AB, Lumsden RM, Swanson GD. Silicone implant arthroplasty of the great toe. A review of single stem and flexible hinge implants. Clin Orthop Relat Res 1979;142:30–43.

105. Shanker NS. Silastic single-stem implants in the treatment of hallux rigidus. Foot Ankle Int 1995;16(8):487–91.

106. Granberry WM, Noble PC, Bishop JO, et al. Use of hinged silicone prosthesis for replacement arthroplasty of the first metatarsophalangeal joint. J Bone Joint Surg Am 1991;73:1453–9.

107. Jarvid BD, Moats DB, Burns A, et al. Lawrence design first metatarsophalangeal joint prosthesis. J Am Podiatr Med Assoc 1986;76:617.

108. Kampner SL. Long-term experience with total joint prosthetic replacement for the arthritic great toe. Bull Hosp Jt Dis Orthop Inst 1987;47:153–77.

109. Konkel KF, Menger AG, Retlaff SA. Results of metallic hemi-great toe implant for grade iii and early grade iv hallux rigidus. Foot Ankle Int 2009;30: 653–60.

110. Sorbie C, Saunders GA. Hemiarthroplasty in the treatment of hallux rigidus. Foot Ankle Int 2008;29:273–81.

111. Maffulli N, Papalia R, Palumbo A, et al. Quantitative review of operative management of hallux rigidus. Br Med Bull 2011;98:75–98.

112. Bonasia DE, Dettoni F, Femino JE, et al. TOTAL ankle replacement: when, why and how? Iowa Orthop J 2010;30:119–30.

113. Saltzman CL, Kadoko RG, Suh JS. Treatment of isolated ankle osteoarthritis with arthrodesis or the total ankle replacement: a comparison of early outcomes. Clin Orthop Surg 2010;2(1):1–7.

114. Ronconi P, Martinelli N, Cancilleri F, et al. Hemiarthroplasty and distal oblique first metatarsal osteotomy for hallux rigidus. Foot Ankle Int 2011;32(2): 148–52.

115. Hasselman CT, Shields N. Resurfacing of the first metatarsal head in the treatment of hallux rigidus. Tech Foot Ankle Surg 2008;7(1):31–40.

116. Konkel KF, Menger AG, Retzlaff SA. Mid-term results of Futura hemi-great toe implants. Foot Ankle Int 2008;29(8):831–7.

117. Konkel KF, Menger AG. Mid-term results of titanium hemi-grade toe implants. Foot Ankle Int 2006;27(11):922–9.

118. Pulavarti RS, McVie JL, Tulloch CJ. First metatarsophalangeal joint replacement using the Bio-Action great toe implant: intermediate results. Foot Ankle Int 2005; 26(12):1033–7.

119. Brewster M. Does total joint replacement or arthrodesis of the first metatarsophalangeal joint yield better functional results? A systematic review of the literature. J Foot Ankle Surg 2010;49(6):546–52.

120. Fuhrmann RA, Wagner A, Anders JO. First metatarsophalangeal joint replacement: the method of choice for end-stage hallux rigidus? Foot Ankle Clin 2003;8(4):711–21.

121. Lapidus PW. The operative correction of the metatarsus primus varus in hallux valgus. Surg Gynecol Obstet 1934;58:183–91.
122. Albrecht GH. The pathology and treatment of hallux valgus. Russ Vrach 1911; 10:14–9.
123. Schenk S, Meizer R, Kramer R, et al. Resection arthroplasty with and without capsular interposition for treatment of severe hallux rigidus. Int Orthop 2009; 33:145–50.
124. Hamilton WE, Hubbard CE. Hallux rigidus. excisional arthroplasty. Foot Ankle Clin 2000;5(3):663–71.
125. Ozan F, Bora OA, Filiz ME, et al. Interposition arthroplasty in the treament of hallux rigidus. Acta Orthop Traumatol Turc 2010;44(2):143–51.
126. Hattrup SJ, Johnson KA. Subjective results of hallux rigidus following treatment with cheilectomy. Clin Orthop 1988;226:182–91.
127. Hyer CF, Granata JD, Berlet GC, et al. Interpositional arthroplasty of the first metatarsophalangeal joint using a regenerative tissue matrix for the treatment of advanced hallux rigidus: 5-year case series follow-up. Foot Ankle Spec 2012;5(4):249–52.
128. DelaCruz EL, Johnson AR, Clair BL. First meratarsophalangeal joint interpositional arthroplasty using a meniscus allograft for the treatment of advanced hallux rigidus: surgical technique and short-term results. Foot Ankle Spec 2011;4(3):157–64.

Revisiting the Tailor's Bunion and Adductovarus Deformity of the Fifth Digit

Lawrence DiDomenico, DPM[a,b,]*, Erigena Baze, DPM[c],
Nikolay Gatalyak, DPM[d]

KEYWORDS

- Tailor's bunion • Adductovaris • Deformity • Fifth digit

KEY POINTS

- Correction of the fifth digit deformity can be rewarding as well as challenging for a foot and ankle surgeon.
- Immense care should be taken when performing any digital procedure, especially of the fifth digits, to avoid and minimize complication rates and mainly to prevent neurovascular damage.

TAILOR'S BUNION
Introduction

Bunionette is a term used to characterize a lateral prominence of the fifth metatarsal head. The term tailor's bunion is also used to refer to this deformity and it is derived from the cross-legged position of a tailor, which places abnormal pressure on the lateral aspect of the fifth metatarsal head.[1–4] Like the bunion, a bunionette has a high association with constrictive shoes.[3,5] The bunionette deformity usually consists of both an abnormal fifth metatarsal as well as overlying soft tissues. The deformities involving the fifth metatarsal and fifth metatarsophalangeal (MTP) joint are characterized by a symptomatic prominence of the fifth metatarsal, which can be accompanied by rotational deformities of the fifth digit. Symptoms can involve the dorsal, lateral, and plantar aspects of the fifth metatarsal head, but most commonly, increased pressure over the lateral condyle of the fifth metatarsal head can lead to chronic irritation of the overlying bursa.[1] Although the incidence and prevalence of tailor's bunionette deformity in the general population is not known, several retrospective studies indicate that

[a] Ankle and Foot Care Centers/Kent State University College of Podiatric Medicine, 6000 Rockside Woods Boulevard Indepedence, OH 44131, USA; [b] St. Elizabeth Medical Center, 8175 Market Street, Youngstown, OH 44512, USA; [c] Heritage Valley Hospital Beaver, Beaver, PA 15108, USA; [d] Private Practice Ankle and Foot Care Centers, 750 E Park Avenue, Columbiana, OH 44408, USA
* Corresponding author.
E-mail address: ld5353@aol.com

Clin Podiatr Med Surg 30 (2013) 397–422
http://dx.doi.org/10.1016/j.cpm.2013.04.004
0891-8422/13/$ – see front matter © 2013 Elsevier Inc. All rights reserved.

the condition is between 3 and 10 times more common in women than men and has a peak incidence during the fourth and fifth decades of life.[6] Conservative treatments such as changes in shoe gear, orthoses, various forms of pressure offloading pads, antiinflammatories, and corticosteroid injections are used in order to lessen the pain associated with a painful tailor's bunionette deformity. However, such modalities have not been shown to provide any long-term relief and merely treat the symptoms associated with the condition and not the deformity itself (**Fig. 1**).[6–8]

Cause

Haskell[9] stated that a bunionette could be considered analogous to the medial eminence of the first metatarsal in hallux valgus. However, the cause and anatomic variations that are present with a bunionette seem to be more complex than those originally described by Kelikian and Davies. Several anatomic factors have been attributed to the development or presence of a bunionette deformity.[10] The bunionette is often seen in splayfoot combined with hallux valgus, or the head of the fifth metatarsal may be congenitally or traumatically enlarged.[11] Also, the shaft may be angulated laterally, making the fifth metatarsal head more prominent.[2,10] Consequently, constricting shoes are the main source of discomfort. With continuous pressure over the prominent fifth metatarsal, a bursa can develop as a result of chronic irritation to the area. Over time, this bursa can develop into an ulceration. In patients with diabetes, advanced Charcot-Marie-Tooth disease, or certain types of spinal dysraphism with poor sensibility, this complication can result in loss of the entire fifth ray or even the foot.[2]

According to Bertrand and colleagues,[1] the cause of bunionette deformities can be divided into 2 broad categories: anatomic and biomechanical.

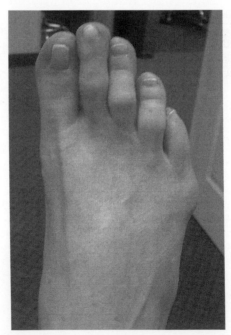

Fig. 1. A patient with a tailor's bunion and a chronic symptomatic irritation of the overlying bursa.

Anatomic causes could include the following:
- Tight footwear causing pressure over the lateral fifth metatarsal
- Abnormal foot position (lateral aspect of the foot resting on the ground)
- Prominent lateral fifth metatarsal head
- Hypertrophy of soft tissues overlying lateral aspect of the fifth metatarsal head
- Dumbbell-shaped fifth metatarsal
- Supernumerary ossicles attached to the lateral fourth metatarsal, pushing the fifth metatarsal laterally
- Increased fourth to fifth intermetatarsal (4–5 IM) angle (splaying)
- Incomplete insertion or development of the transverse metatarsal ligament.

Biomechanical causes could include the following:
- Lateral bending/deviation of the fifth metatarsal
- Congenital plantar or dorsiflexed fifth ray deformities
- Excessive pronation caused by hypermobility of the fifth metatarsal
- Subluxatory pronation of the fifth metatarsal (associated with pronation of subtalar and midtarsal joints)
- Pes planus (hindfoot eversion leads to a more laterally pronounced fifth metatarsal) (**Fig. 2**).

Evaluation

Clinical presentation
The major subjective complaints of a patient presenting with tailor's bunion are pain and irritation caused by friction between the underlying bony abnormality and restricting footwear. Patients complain of swelling, painful ambulation aggravated by shoe gear, and callus formation over the deformity (**Fig. 3**).[12,13]

Classification
Various anatomic variations of the fifth metatarsal have been described in the literature and possible treatment options are based on these variations (see **Fig. 1**A–C). Three

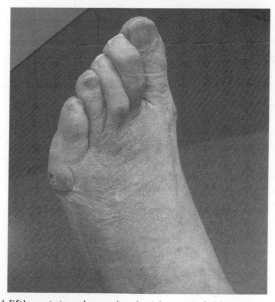

Fig. 2. A deformed fifth metatarsal associated with a painful bursitis.

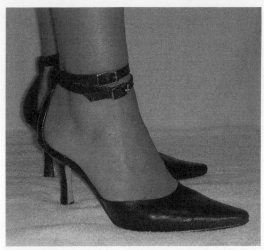

Fig. 3. Constricting shoes, particularly in females, can be a source or a contributing factor in the discomfort of a tailor's bunion.

types of bunionette deformities have been described by Coughlin.[3] The classification is based on weight-bearing dorsoplantar radiographs. In Coughlin's series of symptomatic bunionette deformities, a type I deformity was noted in 27% of cases, a type II deformity in 23% of cases, and type III in 50% of cases.[1,9]

Type I is an enlargement of the lateral surface of the fifth metatarsal. Type I could be secondary to an exostosis; a prominent lateral condyle; or a round, or dumbbell-shaped, metatarsal head. It has been observed that with excessive pronation of the foot, the lateral plantar tubercle of the fifth metatarsal head rotates laterally to create the radiographic impression of an enlarged fifth metatarsal head.

Surgical procedure: a distal osteotomy is the suggested surgical treatment of this deformity (**Fig. 4**).

Type II is secondary to abnormal lateral bowing of the distal fifth metatarsal with a normal 4–5 IM angle. There is not usually associated hypertrophy of the fifth metatarsal head. The bowing of the fifth metatarsal is also called the lateral deviation angle. This angle is formed by 1 line drawn from the center of the fifth metatarsal head to its medial base and a second line made along the medial cortex of the fifth metatarsal. The average lateral deviation angle is normally 2.6° (range, 0°–7°). Symptomatic patients with bunionette deformities have an average value of 8.05° (range, 0°–16°).

Surgical procedure: a diaphyseal or distal osteotomy is the suggested surgical treatment of this deformity (**Fig. 5**).

Type III, the most common in Coughlin's series, is characterized by an increased 4–5 IM angle, with divergence of the fourth and fifth metatarsals.

The average 4–5 IM angle is 6.2° (range 3°–11°). In symptomatic patients with bunionette, the average IM angle is 9.6° (range, 5°–14°).[14,15]

Surgical procedure: a diaphyseal or proximal osteotomy is the suggested surgical treatment of this deformity (**Fig. 6**).

Type IV, not described by Coughlin, is not common and consists of a combination of deformities, including 2 or more of the types listed earlier. This type is most commonly seen in the feet of patients with rheumatoid arthritis.[1]

Although anatomic classification schemes and radiographic criteria are helpful in evaluating and treating bunionette deformities, patients may have increased angles

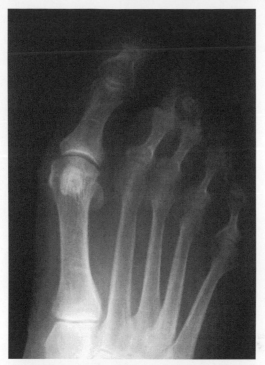

Fig. 4. A patient with a symptomatic enlarged lateral surface of the fifth metatarsal (type I).

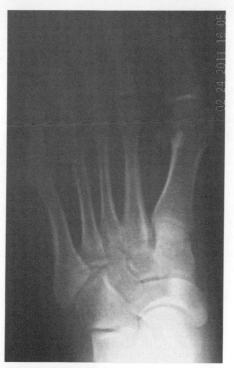

Fig. 5. An anteroposterior radiograph showing an abnormal lateral bowing of the distal fifth metatarsal with a normal 4–5 IM angle (type II).

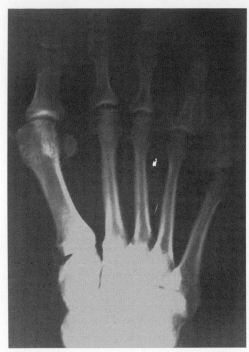

Fig. 6. An anteroposterior radiograph showing an increased IM angle with divergence of the fourth and fifth metatarsal heads.

and no symptoms, or patients may have more than 1 anatomic variation, complicating decision making. In addition, with pronation of the foot, the 4–5 IM angle was found to increase by 3°, and the fifth metatarsal head appears to increase in size, suggesting that radiographic technique may influence significantly preoperative and postoperative assessment.[10]

Regardless of the underlying anatomy, the common symptom that all patients with a bunionette deformity note is increased pressure over the fifth metatarsal head caused by constricting footwear. This symptom seems more exaggerated in the female population because of choices in fashionable shoe gear. Swelling of the soft tissues overlying the lateral aspect of the fifth metatarsal head can lead to pain. Three main painful areas that have been described in relation to the head of fifth metatarsal are laterally, dorsolaterally, and plantarly. Patients with a bunionette deformity often present with erythema and edema over a deformity on the lateral aspect of the foot. In immunocompromised patients, ulceration can occur, which can lead to superinfection. Over time, as continuous pressure is applied over the lateral aspect of the fifth metatarsal, a secondary hyperkeratotic lesion can develop over the lateral or plantar aspects of the fifth toe. This hyperkeratosis can occasionally cause the fifth toe to deviate medially at the MTP joint, whereas the metatarsal deviates laterally (**Figs. 7–9**).[1]

Radiographic evaluation
Tailor's bunion deformity can be evaluated with plain foot weight-bearing radiographs. Anteroposterior (AP) and lateral radiographs are the standard views used to evaluate the deformity. Occasionally, a medial oblique (MO) view is performed to assess lateral flare, metatarsal head, lateral tubercle, and lateral soft tissues. The most common

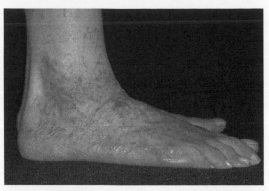

Fig. 7. A clinical view of a patient with dorsal lateral tailor's bunion pain.

radiographic angles used to evaluate tailor's bunion deformity are the 4–5 IM angle and lateral deviation angle.

The 4–5 IM angle measures the divergence of the respective metatarsal and can be achieved by the traditional method, bisecting the shafts of the fourth and fifth metatarsals. An alternative measurement to evaluate the divergence is using a line drawn along the medial and proximal border of the fifth metatarsal and bisection of the fourth metatarsal. According to Fallat and Buckholz,[14] the average IM angle using the traditional method is 6.2°, with a range of 3° to 11°, although in their study, the average

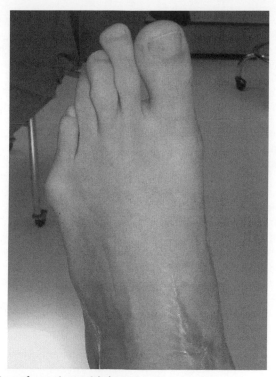

Fig. 8. A clinical view of a patient with lateral tailor's bunion pain.

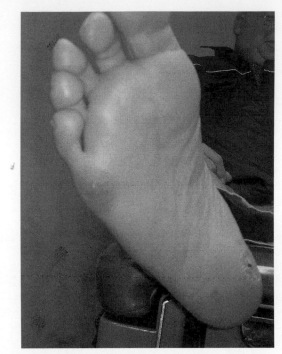

Fig. 9. A clinical view of a patient with plantar fifth metatarsal callus, causing pain.

angle in a symptomatic tailor's bunion deformity was 9.6° and may be increased an average of 3° in patients with pes planus deformity.

As the IM angle increases, more pressure is shown on the lateral metatarsal head, and the same can be observed with lateral deviation angle. The lateral deviation angle is a measurement of a line bisecting the metatarsal head and neck and a line drawn along the medial and proximal border of the metatarsal cortex. Fallat and Buckholz found the average angle in a normal foot to be 2.64° and 8.05° in patients with tailor's bunion deformity.

Physical examination

Emphasis is placed on evaluation of the foot and ankle for presence of adventitial bursa formations, keratotic lesions, and ulcerations. In addition, according to Roukis and colleagues,[6] a detailed evaluation of the fifth metatarsal cuboid joint and fifth metatarsal phalangeal joint range of motion, global forefoot posture, and palpation of the periarticular structures to determine areas of maximum signs and symptoms and exostosis formation should be performed.

The clinical examination should include a through assessment of the patient's past and present medical history, with special emphasis placed on the chronicity of the symptoms, effect of the condition on their activities of daily living and employment responsibilities, and progression of the deformity.

However, weight-bearing radiographs are essential, and when combined with the clinical examination, allow complete evaluation in all but the most severe or unusual abnormalities involving the fifth metatarsal and fifth metatarsal phalangeal joint. Weight-bearing AP and lateral radiographs in the angle and base of gait should be made of both feet if disease exists bilateral or of the symptomatic foot, with any necessary comparison views of the contralateral uninvolved foot to allow for full evaluation of the structural alignment and osseous morphology of the forefoot and specifically the fifth metatarsal.

Treatment Options

Nonsurgical management

Conservative treatment should be aimed toward patient education of the deformity in order to increase compliance. Proper-fitting shoe gear is essential, because many of the patient's symptoms can arise from placing increased pressure on the lateral foot and fifth metatarsal head, thus irritating the overlying skin and capsule; swelling of the fifth metatarsal bursa may also occur.[2,5] Extra depth shoes or tennis shoes with a wider toe box can decrease direct pressure and improve symptoms. In addition, leather-style shoes may be stretched over the painful prominence by a podorthist.[1,2,4,5,16,17]

The use of oral antiinflammatory medication and local corticosteroid injections in an inflamed bursa may reduce local tissue inflammation.[4,17]

In cases in which the prominent metatarsal head is accompanied by hyperkeratotic lesion, debridement and padding should be performed. When pain over the fifth metatarsal head is caused by abnormal foot mechanics, prefabricated or custom orthotics may be used to alleviate symptoms and decrease pronation of the subtalar joint.

Surgical management

Operative management is warranted in patients with symptomatic bunionette deformity who have not responded to nonsurgical treatment. This management may also be the line of approach for patients with special demands, such as high-performing athletes. The procedure performed is dictated by the anatomic and biomechanical findings made during the preoperative evaluation.

The goals of surgical intervention are to decrease the width of the forefoot as well as the prominence of the bunionette. Correction of the underlying disease is necessary to prevent a recurrence of the deformity. Likewise, preservation of function of the fifth MTP joint may prevent such complications as recurrence, subluxation, dislocation, or the development of a transfer lesion.[1]

Osteotomy Techniques

Operative procedures can be divided into exostectomies, resections, and various metatarsal osteotomies.[2] Metatarsal osteotomies can be divided based on the anatomic location: proximal, diaphyseal, or distal. Other options that have been described but are of limited usefulness are metatarsal head resection, fifth metatarsal ray resection, and isolated soft tissue procedures.

Head procedures

Lateral condyle resection Partial resection of the lateral condyle of the fifth metatarsal head is probably the most commonly used procedure. This procedure has been termed an ostectomy, exostectomy, condylectomy, or simple bunionectomy and can be performed in isolation or as part of other surgical techniques.[6,7] It relieves the pressure symptoms and allows a slightly greater variety of shoe wear.[2]

The use of this technique as an isolated procedure was initially advocated by Davies in 1949.[6] It is indicated to correct hypertrophy of the dorsal or lateral aspect of the fifth metatarsal head region without soft tissue or structural deformity and when more aggressive or involved procedures are not appropriate for the patient.[6]

Kitaoka and Holiday[18] reported 15 good results, 3 fair results, and 3 poor results in 21 feet treated with lateral condylar resection for painful bunionettes. Causes of failure were inadequate resection, MTP joint subluxation, and forefoot splaying. Therefore, the patient must be warned before surgery that only the painful bony prominence will be removed, and no other preexisting conditions such as the width of the forefoot will change with this procedure. In addition, if there is a painful callosity beneath the metatarsal head, the plantar aspect of the condyle also should be removed.[2]

Surgical technique[9]
- Center a longitudinal skin incision over the lateral condyle of the fifth metatarsal.
- Protect the dorsal cutaneous nerve of the fifth toe.
- Create an inverted L-type capsular incision by detaching the dorsal and proximal capsular attachments, allowing exposure of the fifth metatarsal head.
- Distract the fifth MTP joint and release the medial capsule.
- Resect the lateral eminence with an osteotome or sagittal saw.
- Close the MTP capsule by suturing it to the dorsal periosteum and to the abductor digiti quinti proximally.
- If necessary, place a suture through a drill hole in the fifth metatarsal metaphysic dorsal and lateral to ensure a stable capsular closure and prevent recurrence or lateral subluxation of the MTP joint.

Resection of fifth metatarsal head Excision of the fifth metatarsal head, resection of the distal half of the metatarsal, and fifth ray resection have all been used to treat a bunionette deformity but are not appropriate in the initial treatment of symptomatic conditions (**Fig. 10**).[9]

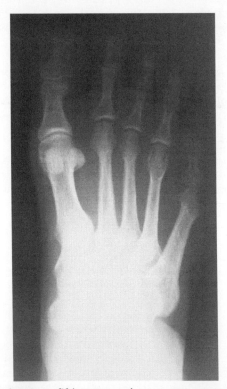

Fig. 10. AP radiograph showing a fifth metatarsal ostectomy, exostectomy, condylectomy, or simple bunionectomy. We caution that this procedure can be associated with causing a degree of instability at the fifth metatarsal phalangeal joint.

Surgical technique (Ishiwaka)
- Make a midlateral incision over the distal third of the metatarsal to expose the metatarsal head, and remove it obliquely 5 mm proximal to the capsular insertion at the head-neck junction.
- Close the capsule with absorbable sutures and the skin with nonabsorbable sutures.

Kitaoka and Holiday[18] reported poor results in 7 of 11 feet with metatarsal head resection; 2 had fair results, and only 2 had good results at an average follow-up of 9 years. Causes of failure were transfer metatarsalgia, persistent lateral forefoot prominence, and painful fifth toe deformity.[2] These investigators did not recommend this procedure for initial operative treatment of bunionette deformity.

Dorris and Mandel[19] performed a retrospective review of 50 such procedures in 34 patients for severe, recurring keratotic lesions to the plantar aspect of the fifth metatarsal head. They reported a 59% incidence of fifth digit malalignment, and Addante and colleagues[9,20] reported malalignment and wound problems after metatarsal head resection and silicone implant arthroplasty.

Therefore, this procedure is considered unstable and is used as a salvage procedure for infection, ulceration, or severe deformity. Situations in which this procedure may be appropriate include severe osteopenia, extensive degenerative joint changes, chronic ulceration with or without osteomyelitis, previous failed surgery, or poor medical health (**Fig. 11**).[6,8,9]

Distal metatarsal osteotomies
Chevron osteotomy Following the success of a stable construct for the Austin (chevron) hallux bunionectomy, many investigators such as Kitaoka used a similar technique for the bunionette deformity as well.[16,21] In their series, these investigators reported pain relief in 15 of a total of 19 patients. Two patients required revision surgery because of severe residual pain. The 4-5 IM angle was reduced an average of 2.6°, and the MTP5 angle was reduced an average of 8° with the chevron osteotomy.

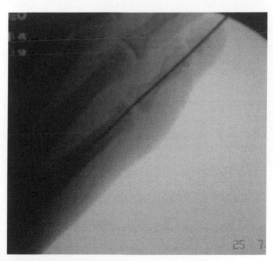

Fig. 11. An intraoperative radiograph showing a distal metatarsal resection with K-wire fixation. We caution that there is a great instability at the metatarsal phalangeal joint associated with this type of procedure.

Although the investigators believed that the osteotomy was stable, they used internal fixation with a short threaded Kirschner wire. With the dorsally directed force of weight bearing in line with the osteotomy, excess dorsal displacement is possible without internal fixation. If fixation is not performed, there may be increased risk of transfer metatarsalgia.[22]

Moran and Claridge stressed that there was a low margin of error with this osteotomy and that there was a high risk for either recurrence or overcorrection. As a result, these investigators encouraged the use of Kirschner wire stabilization of the osteotomy site.[9,22]

Surgical technique (Haskell)

- Make a midlateral longitudinal incision over the lateral eminence.
- Release the proximal and dorsal capsule using an L-type capsular incision.
- Avoid soft tissue stripping to avoid vascular insult to the distal metatarsal fragment.
- Remove about 2 mm of the lateral eminence with an osteotome or a sagittal saw.
- Mark the apex of the osteotomy with a drill hole in the midportion of the metatarsal.
- Create a horizontal chevron osteotomy with a sagittal saw. The osteotomy is based proximally with an angle of 60° and oriented in a lateral to medial direction (**Fig. 12**).
- Displace the distal fragment about 2 to 3 mm in a medial direction and impacted onto the proximal phalanx.
- Use Kirschner wire fixation when necessary.
- Remove any remaining prominent bone in the metaphyseal region of the fifth metatarsal with a sagittal saw.
- Reef the lateral capsule of the fifth metatarsal. If necessary, reattach the capsule through drill holes on the dorsal aspect of the metaphysis.

Distal oblique osteotomy   Helal originally described the osteotomy in 1975 for treatment of intractable plantar keratosis. The osteotomy as originally described sloped in a dorsal proximal to a plantar distal direction at a 45° angle. The original description mentioned no internal fixation and immediate weight bearing.[23]

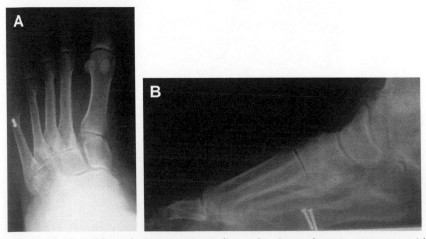

Fig. 12. (*A*, *B*) AP and lateral postoperative radiograph using a chevron osteotomy with 2 dorsal-plantar cortical screws.

According to Fiebel, Pedowitz reported one of the few positive results of the Helal osteotomy without internal fixation. A total of 41 of the 49 procedures had a good or excellent rating. Three patients had transfer lesions and 2 had nonunions, both of which were asymptomatic.

In addition, Winson and colleagues performed the metatarsal osteotomy as described by Helal. Of 124 feet, 63 had metatarsal head prominence and callosities postoperatively. Twenty-seven feet had malunions of the osteotomy site. The following factors were identified as predisposing to a poor result: patient age greater than 65 years, postoperative plaster of Paris immobilization, and poor lesser toe function.[23]

Weil originally described an osteotomy that is currently popular. This osteotomy is often compared with the Helal osteotomy in the literature. However, a review of the literature shows better results with the Weil osteotomy compared with the Helal. The Weil osteotomy allows for a more predictable amount of shortening. The results have also improved with stable internal fixation. Most of the reports on the Helal osteotomy do not use internal fixation.[23]

Surgical technique (Haskell)
- Make a midlateral longitudinal incision over the lateral eminence.
- Release the proximal and dorsal capsule using an L-type capsular incision.
- Release the abductor digiti quinti and resect the lateral eminence with an osteotome or sagittal saw.
- Create the oblique osteotomy of the metaphyseal neck using either a saw or an osteotome. The osteotomy is oriented in a proximal lateral to distal medial direction.
- Displace the distal fragment medially on the metatarsal and impact the bone on the proximal fragment.

Metatarsal neck osteotomy Distal fifth metatarsal head-neck osteotomies are considered efficacious for correction of mild to moderate transverse and sagittal plane deformities.[6,7]

Hohman originally described a transverse osteotomy of the metatarsal neck. The lack of stability of this procedure increases the risk for a transfer lesion or a malunion.[9]

Metatarsal shaft osteotomies
The indications for a diaphyseal fifth metatarsal osteotomy are a bunionette deformity associated with either an increased 4-5 IM angle or lateral bowing of the distal metatarsal.[9]

Voutey carried out a transverse osteotomy in the diaphysis but described problems with rotation, angulation, and pseudarthrosis.

Oblique diaphyseal osteotomy A long, oblique, diaphyseal osteotomy of the fifth metatarsal for severe splayfoot or metatarsus quintus valgus can correct a great degree of deformity. The incidence of delayed union/nonunion is more common than with distal metaphyseal head osteotomies. However, Coughlin[3] reported good or excellent results in 93% feet treated with longitudinal diaphyseal osteotomy, lateral condylectomy, and distal metatarsal joint soft tissue realignment.

Surgical technique (Coughlin)
- Make a longitudinal incision centered on the dorsolateral aspect of the fifth metatarsal extending from the base of the fifth metatarsal to the middle of the proximal phalanx. Protect the dorsolateral cutaneous nerve during dissection.

- Reflect the abductor digiti quinti muscle plantarward to expose the fifth metatarsal diaphysis. Leave the soft tissue attachments to the medial aspect intact.
- Expose the MTP joint capsule, and make an L-shaped incision along the dorsal and proximal aspects to expose the lateral eminence.
- After the capsule is detached, use a sagittal saw to resect the lateral condyle of the metatarsal head.
- Distract the MTP joint by applying distal traction to the fifth toe, and release the medial capsule of the MTP joint so that it can be realigned after the osteotomy is made.
- Use a sagittal saw to make an osteotomy in the fifth metatarsal diaphysis. For pure lateral keratosis, direct the cut from lateral to medial, with the obliquity oriented from a dorsal- proximal to a plantar distal direction. If plantar and lateral keratoses are present, angle the saw blade slightly upward to elevate the fifth metatarsal head. For a pure plantar keratosis, when more elevation of the distal fragment is desired, increase the obliquity of the osteotomy.
- Before completing the osteotomy, drill fixation holes in the proximal and distal fragments. Because the diaphysis is so narrow, placement of the holes after osteotomy can be difficult.
- Complete the osteotomy and rotate the distal fragment medially so that it is parallel with the fourth metatarsal, using the fixation hole as the axis for rotation. It is important that the osteotomy is rotated rather than translated to ensure maximal bony contact; rotation also maintains metatarsal length.
- Fix the osteotomy with a small fragment screw, screw and Kirschner wire, or multiple Kirschner wires.
- Realign the fifth toe by reefing the lateral capsule to the fifth metatarsal metaphyseal periosteum and the abductor digiti quinti. If tissue is insufficient to attach the MTP capsule, place interrupted sutures through holes drilled in the metaphysis. This capsular plication allows significant correction of axial malalignment or malrotation.

Coughlin's study reported on 30 feet that had undergone a midshaft diaphyseal metatarsal osteotomy, all of which went on to successful union. The average 4–5 IM angle was reduced 10°, and the MTP5 angle was reduced 16°. The average foot width was reduced 6 mm and no transfer lesions developed.

Vienne and colleagues reported good or excellent results in 97% of their series of patients with diaphyseal osteotomies for bunionette correction. In this study, the 4–5 IM angle was reduced from an average of 10° preoperatively to 1° postoperatively.[24]

Castle and colleagues reported a retrospective review of 26 long oblique wedge resection osteotomies. These investigators found a mean 4–5 IM angle reduction of 1.58° (7.9°–6.48°) and a mean lateral deviation angle reduction of 3.98° (4.1°–0.28°). One osteotomy fractured after a traumatic incident in the early postoperative period, but there were no reported incidences of delayed union, malunion, or transfer lesions.[25]

Base Osteotomy

Closing base wedge osteotomy

Proximal osteotomies are associated with a higher incidence of nonunion secondary to potential injury to the blood supply to the fifth metatarsal.[9]

Proximal fifth metatarsal base osteotomies are used to reduce increased 4–5 IM angles. The osteotomy configurations described include closing and opening base wedges, crescent-shaped in the sagittal and transverse planes. However, the vascular supply in the proximal base region at the metaphyseal-diaphyseal junction, where the osteotomies are commonly performed, minimizes the use of this procedure.

Surgical technique (Chao)

- Use a dorsal approach to expose the metatarsal head. Make a longitudinal incision in the capsule, and debride the joint, removing loose fragments. Perform a partial synovectomy.
- Make a dorsal closing wedge osteotomy over the distal normal metaphysis, removing sufficient bone to bring the healthy plantar part of the metatarsal head into articulation with the phalanx.
- Do not remove the lesion, but rotate it proximally and dorsally.
- The angle of the closing wedge should maintain the length of the involved metatarsal bone as much as possible.
- Temporarily fix the osteotomy with crossed percutaneous Kirschner wires.

Gerbert and colleagues[26] described a preliminary report on the use of a closing base wedge osteotomy to the fifth metatarsal in 20 feet with favorable results.

Diebold performed a retrospective review of 22 proximal fifth metatarsal base chevron osteotomies fixated with several horizontally oriented Kirschner wires between the fifth and fourth metatarsals. There was a minimum follow-up period of 3 years. The mean 4–5 IM angle reduction was 10.88° (12.1° –1.38°), with no incidence of nonunion, malunion, or transfer lesions. The investigators concluded that the significant stability caused by transmetatarsal pinning over crossed fixation of the osteotomy was responsible for the lack of malunions and nonunions experienced in their studies.[27]

Preferred Techniques for Tailor's Bunion

We believe the best correction for a tailor's bunion is to perform the osteotomy at the level of the deformity in the fifth metatarsal. In addition, it has been our experience that if the deformity is corrected at the appropriate site, it is not necessary to enter into the fifth metatarsal phalangeal joint. Advantages of not entering the fifth metatarsal phalangeal joint are many: maintenance of the articular surface; the fifth metatarsal phalangeal joint cannot get stiff; there is no staking of the metatarsal head; there is no instability to the fifth metatarsal phalangeal joint; and there is no neuritis associated with the procedure at the metatarsal phalangeal joint.

Distal metatarsal osteotomy

A dorsal lateral incision is made over the distal one-third of the fifth metatarsal. The incision is carried down to the bone, avoiding neurovascular structures. An oblique corrective osteotomy is made at the level of the deformity, with the base being medial and the apex being lateral. The lateral cortex is left intact, and bone resection is performed until the deformity is reduced and the metatarsal phalangeal joint is well aligned. Next, temporary fixation is applied, and a multiple-hole locking plate is applied laterally, with interfragmentary compression through the plate. A locking plate is used in cases in which we want to provide immediate weight bearing with a protective walking boot (**Fig. 13**).

Midshaft osteotomy

A dorsal lateral incision is made over the midshaft of the fifth metatarsal. The incision is carried down to the bone, avoiding neurovascular structures. An oblique corrective osteotomy is made at the level of the deformity, with the base being medial and the apex being lateral. The lateral cortex is left intact, and bone resection is performed until

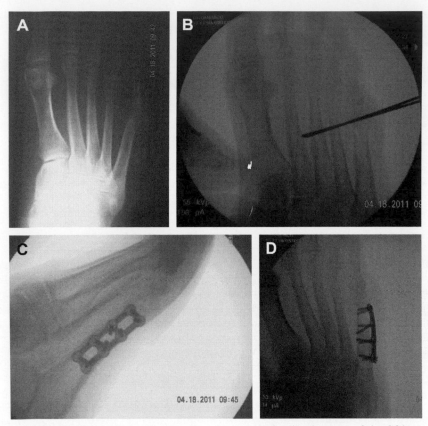

Fig. 13. (*A*) AP radiograph showing a tailor's bunion at the distal aspect of the fifth meta-tarsal. (*B*) An intraoperative radiograph showing the osteotomy was performed at the level of the deformity within the fifth metatarsal and temporary reduced with K-wire fixation. (*C*) A lateral intraoperative radiograph showing a multiple-hole locking plate with stacked screws, providing more resistance to ground reactive forces with early weight bearing. (*D*) Intraoperative radiograph showing a multiple-hole locking plate. Please note that the os-teotomy is reduced with an interfragmentary compression screw through the locking plate.

the deformity is reduced and the metatarsal phalangeal joint is well aligned. Next, tem-porary fixation is applied, and a multiple-hole locking plate is applied laterally, with inter-fragmentary compression through the plate. A locking plate is used in cases in which we want to provide immediate weight bearing with a protective walking boot (**Fig. 14**).

Base osteotomy

A dorsal lateral incision is made over the proximal shaft of the fifth metatarsal. The inci-sion is carried down to the bone, avoiding neurovascular structures. An oblique corrective osteotomy is made at the level of the deformity, with the base being medial and the apex being lateral. The lateral cortex is left intact, and bone resection is per-formed until the deformity is reduced to the point at which the IM angle is almost par-allel and the metatarsal phalangeal joint is well aligned. Next, temporary fixation is applied, and a multiple-hole locking plate is applied laterally, with interfragmentary compression through the plate. A locking plate is used in cases in which we want to provide immediate weight bearing with a protective walking boot (**Fig. 15**).

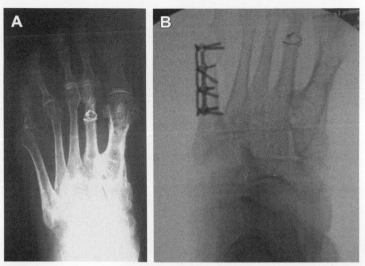

Fig. 14. (*A*) A preoperative AP radiograph showing a midshaft deformity with subluxation of the fifth metatarsal phalangeal joint. (*B*) An intraoperative radiograph showing reduction of the 4–5 IM angle. Note the metatarsal phalangeal joint reduction achieved by performing the osteotomy at the level of the deformity.

Complications

Pain and recurrence after surgical correction are mostly caused by incorrect procedure being chosen in order to address the deformity. Also, patients who underwent metatarsal head resection were more likely to experience pain sub fourth metatarsal head and concomitant underlying transfer lesion compared with other corrective procedures. Flail fifth toe may also be observed with this type of procedure, and syndactylization to the fourth digit may be required. After performing distal metatarsal procedures, subluxation of the MTP joint can occur. This complication can be avoided by tight and meticulous closure and repair of the lateral capsule.

Improper soft tissue handling and excessive soft tissue stripping can cause avascular necrosis of the metatarsal head or delayed union or nonunion at the osteotomy site. Proximal metatarsal osteotomies are at greater risk than distal osteotomies of having delayed union or nonunion because of blood supply and the unstable nature of proximal osteotomies. Delayed union is considered when an average rate of healing is not achieved for a period of 3 to 6 months.[28] Nonunion is established when bone union is not seen for 6 to 9 months, with no visible progression of healing for 3 months.[28,29] This situation is typically seen when excessive motion occurs at the fracture or osteotomy site secondary to unprotected weight bearing or inadequate or poor fixation placement, which can also so lead to distraction at the osteotomy site and loss of surgical correction; malunion can result.[30,31]

Summary

A variety of conservative treatments and surgical osteotomy procedures have been described in the literature for the bunionette deformity. We recommend making the correction at the level of the deformity and reducing the osteotomies close to normal anatomic alignment. In addition, we suggest not entering the metatarsal phalangeal joint, which should lead to a decline in complications. Utilization of locking plates allows patients to ambulate early with a protective boot.

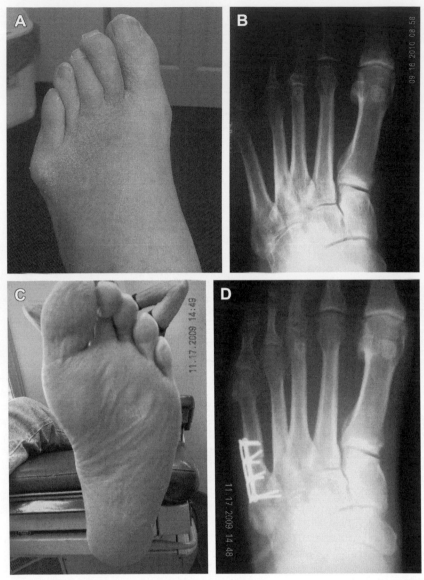

Fig. 15. (*A, B*) A clinical and radiographic preoperative view of a patient with a tailor's bunion with an increase in the 4–5 IM angle. (*C, D*) A clinical and radiograph postoperative view after a base osteotomy fixated with a multiple-hole locking plate. Note the reduction of the 4–5 IM angle.

Metatarsal osteotomies narrow the forefoot, maintain the length of the metatarsal, and preserve function of the MTP joint.[21] Fifth metatarsal osteotomies are categorized into distal, midshaft, and base osteotomies. Distal metatarsal osteotomies produce less correction. Diaphyseal osteotomies are indicated when greater correction is needed and the 4–5 IM angle needs to be addressed. Proximal base osteotomies may be used to address significantly increased 4-5 IM angles or when a large degree of sagittal plane correction is required.

Postoperatively, early protective weight bearing, low-profile internal fixation, and protection of the surrounding soft tissue supportive structures should be used to ensure a successful outcome with minimal complications, if allowed by the level and fixation techniques.[6–8]

ADDUCTOVARUS FIFTH DIGIT
Introduction

The contracture of the digits is known as hammer toe deformity or hammer digit syndrome.[32,33] These digital deformities can be divided into 3 types: hammer toe, claw toe, and mallet toe.[17,32,34]

Cause

The hammer toe deformity is the most common type of digital deformity. It occurs mostly in the sagittal plane, where the MTP joint is extended, the proximal interphalangeal joint is flexed, and the distal interphalangeal joint is extended.[32,33] Claw toe deformity is similar in appearance to hammer toe, with the exception of the flexion contracture of the distal interphalangeal joint, and mallet toe deformity is identified by flexion contracture of the distal interphalangeal joint alone.[32,33]

The 3 main causes of hammer toe syndrome are flexor stabilization, flexor substitution, and extensor substitution. Flexor stabilization is considered the most common cause of hammer toe deformity and occurs mainly in flexible flatfoot deformity, in which there is abnormal subtalar joint pronation.[32,35,36] It leads to unlocking of the midtarsal joint, allowing it to become hypermobile. This event allows the flexors to gain mechanical advantage over the interosseous muscles attempting to stabilize the hypermobile foot, causing reverse buckling of the digits and resulting in a contracture deformity.[36,37] Through these events, the quadratus plantae muscle becomes less effective because of the change in direction of force caused by the flexor digitorum longus.[37] The pull of the flexor digitorum longus is now more proximal and medial, creating a frontal plane rotation of the digits, which gives rise to the adductovarus deformity. The fifth digit is affected more than the fourth and even the third digits because of increase in medial pull of the flexor digitorum longus tendon on the fifth digit versus the third. Peripheral neuropathy is another reason why interosseous muscles can become weakened, leading to similar digital contractures.[32,38]

Flexor substitution is the least common cause of a hammer toe deformity. It is observed mostly in the supinated foot type, in which there is a weak triceps surae muscle. The long flexors aid in plantarflexion of the ankle, producing digital contracture because of its mechanical advantage over the interossei muscles. As this occurs, adductovarus contracture is unlikely compared with flexor stabilization, because of its supinated foot type.[32]

Extensor substitution also causes digital contractures, although they mainly occur in the swing phase of gait. Extensor substitution mostly occurs in the cavus or supinated foot type, in which the extensor digitorum longus tendon gains mechanical advantage over the lumbricales.[32,36–38] Clinically, bowstringing of the extensor tendons and claw toe digital contractures are commonly seen.

Evaluation

Clinical presentation
Patients mostly present with the main complaint of painful digital deformity.[39] Frontal plane rotation and adduction of the digit can be seen in addition to the contracture of the interphalangeal joints. MTP joint extension is not uncommon with adductovarus hammer toe deformity (**Fig. 16**).

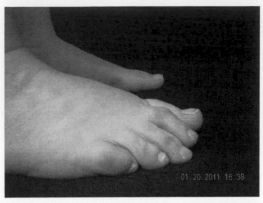

Fig. 16. A clinical view of an adductovarus deformity of the fifth digit.

Because of the rotated nature of the digit, a Lister corn in the lateral nail groove can be thick and painful.[40] Also thickening and dystrophy of the nail is common because of irritation by shoe gear. Hyperkeratotic lesions can develop from direct pressure of the bony prominences between the fourth and fifth digits.[40] A lesion can also be noted on the dorsolateral proximal interphalangeal joint caused by shoe pressure on the digit **(Fig. 17)**.[13]

Radiographic evaluation
Radiographic evaluation is most commonly performed with standard AP, MO, and lateral views of the weight-bearing foot.[12,17] Commonly, the fusion of the distal and middle phalangeal bones can be seen on all 3 views.[32] Lesion markers can be used to evaluate location of painful lesions and assess the location and extent of bony deformity as well.

Physical examination
Physical examination should begin by evaluating the vascular status of the lower extremity. This examination is crucial in the decision-making process in order to attempt surgical correction. Patients with vascular compromise can also have a significant amount of pain from lack of oxygen to the digit. Ulcerations and local soft tissue

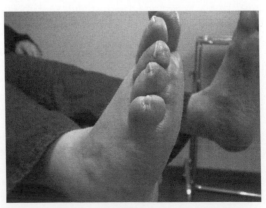

Fig. 17. A clinical view of a patient who suffers from a Lister's corn.

infection as a result of untreated hyperkeratotic lesions can complicate the outcome and change the treatment regimen.

The examiner should perform a musculoskeletal evaluation, paying close attention to any muscle group weakness or overpowering, limited joint range of motion, hypermobility of joints, and osseous foot deformity. The evaluation should also be performed while the patient is ambulating. The patient's neurologic status should also be assessed for neuropathy which can lead to intrinsic muscle weakness and produce digital deformity.

Treatment Options

Nonsurgical management

The main goal of conservative treatment of adductovarus hammer toe deformity is to decrease direct pressure and shearing forces on the digit. Initially, this goal can be achieved by wearing wider shoes with a higher toe box.[35,39,41,42] Bony prominences and hyperkeratotic lesions can be padded with foam or gel toe sleeves. Aperture pads and toe spacers can also give pain relief and offload painful dorsal and interdigital lesions.[13,41] Debridement of the hyperkeratotic lesions alleviates pressure and pain of the digit.[41] Strengthening exercises of the intrinsic musculature can be helpful early in the deformity process by practicing grabbing small objects with the toes (**Fig. 18**).[13]

Surgical management

Condylectomy Contracture and frontal plane rotation deformity of the fifth digits can be painful in the presence of hyperkeratotic lesions overlying bony prominences. The lesions are usually present on the proximal phalanx medial or lateral as well as lateral to the distal phalanx.[25] Attempting to resolve the underlying pressure point may be beneficial in relieving pain.

This procedure is performed through a dorsal linear incision, and the prominent condyle or condyles are exposed and resected with bone rongeurs or power instrumentation and rasped smooth at the end.[40] This is a simple procedure with quick recovery and minimal complications.

Arthroplasty Digital arthroplasty is one of the most common procedures used to correct hammer toe deformity. It involves resection of the proximal phalangeal head, resulting in relaxation of the long flexor tendon.

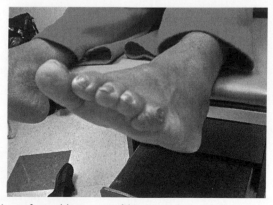

Fig. 18. A clinical view of an adductovarus fifth digit after a debridement of hyperkeratosis.

Typically, this procedure is achieved by a dorsal linear incision over the proximal interphalangeal head,[40] although it is not uncommon for the incision to be extended more proximally to gain access to the MTP joint in order to perform a capsular release of the contracted joint. In addition, an extensor hood release and Z-tendon lengthening can be performed to help reduce the contracture deformity. Kirschner wire can be used to provide stability across the interphalangeal joints as well as the metatarsophalangeal joint, maintaining correct alignment of the digit during the postoperative period.[40]

The wire is usually left in place for a period of 4 to 6 weeks, allowing for fibrosis to occur, and the digit should be kept in the correct position once the wire is removed. Depending on the severity of the digital adductovarus rotation, this procedure alone may not fully correct the frontal plane deformity. A derotational skin plasty should be considered (**Fig. 19**).

Skin plasty Skin plasty of the fifth digits is a great adjunctive procedure for correction of varus or frontal plane deformity, but it is rarely used alone. Although uncommon, it can be performed solely to excise deep-seated calluses and provide substantial pain relief.

When performing a derotational skin plasty, clinical and radiographic evaluation should be performed to identify the apex of the contracture deformity so that it can be properly addressed. Most commonly, the apex of the deformity is located at the proximal interphalangeal joint, but it can also be seen at the distal interphalangeal joint, thus requiring a middle phalangectomy procedure.

The derotational skin plasty is achieved by making 2 semielliptical incisions on the dorsal aspect of the digit.[41] Typically, they are obliquely oriented from distal medial and extending to proximal lateral over the proximal interphalangeal joint. The skin wedge excised can also encompass a symptomatic dorsal hyperkeratosis.[40,31] Care should be exercised when performing the incision to avoid neurovascular structures. Once the procedure is complete, the digit is helped into the corrected position and skin closure is then performed.[40,41]

Syndactyly Syndactyly of the fourth to fifth digits is not commonly performed as a primary procedure. Mostly, it is used in cases in which previous surgery was attempted

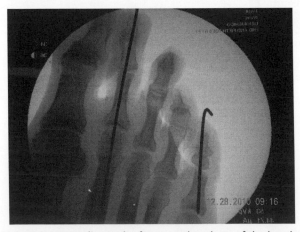

Fig. 19. An intraoperative AP radiograph after an arthroplasty of the head of the fifth proximal phalanx with K-wire fixation.

to correct the deformity but failed, leaving patients with an unstable, flail fifth digit.[39] It has been reported that this procedure has also been used in surgical treatment of interdigital corn.[40] The main goal is to achieve a stable fifth digit.

This goal is achieved by marking the medial side of the fifth digit and compressing the fourth and fifth toes together. The mark should leave a mirror image on the fourth toe.[43] Then a full-thickness skin excision is carried out. The 2 toes are sutured together and given adequate healing time.

Amputation Amputation is considered the last option when previous surgical attempts to correct the deformity have been unsuccessful.[39,40] It is also the procedure used when surgical complications arise, such as deep infection, osteomyelitis, or gangrene.[40]

Preferred Technique for Adductovarus Deformity

We recommend noninvasive vascular examination of those patients who may be at risk for vascular compromise. We have excellent experience with performing flexor digitorum longus–fifth tendon transfer as the surgical treatment of choice.

The flexor digitorum longus–fifth tendon transfer is performed as a medial approach midline incision of the fifth digit. The incision is carried deep to the deep fascia, avoiding neurovascular structures. The deep fascia tissue is incised, and the flexor digitorum longus tendon is identified. The flexor digitorum longus tendon is traced as far proximal to the web space and as far distal to its attachment on the base of the distal phalanx. The tendon is detached from the base of the distal phalanx, allowing the adductor pull and flexor contracture to be released. The flexor digitorum brevis (both the medial and lateral heads) is detached from the base of the middle phalanx. This procedure also reduces any remaining flexion contracture. Next, if necessary, a capsulotomy is performed at the proximal or distal interphalangeal joint to obtain a full reduction of any remaining contracture. A 15.75-mm (0.62-inch) K-wire is inserted from the distal phalanx through the distal and proximal interphalangeal joint, ensuring complete reduction of the flexor and adductor contracture. With the fifth digit in the desired position, the flexor digitorum longus tendon is then transferred to the extensor hood on the medial dorsal aspect of the fifth toe. The toe is put into the desired anatomic position and physiologic tension is applied to the tendon as it is sutured

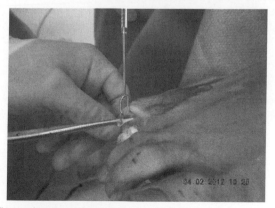

Fig. 20. The fifth flexor digitorum longus tendon is released from the midline medial incision. A gauze sponge is used to wrap around the fourth digit to retract it from the surgical field.

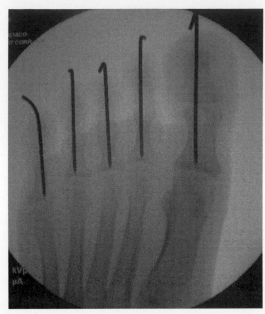

Fig. 21. An intraoperative photograph after flexor digitorum longus tendon transfer performed for adductovarus deformity of a fifth toe as well as flexor contractures of digits 1 to 5.

to the extensor hood. The skin is closed in typical fashion. The K-wire is removed in 7 days, and the sutures are removed at 14 days.

We have experienced advantages such as less postoperative edema, the length of time the K-wire fixation is needed, surgical cosmesis (medial interdigital incision), and the surgical procedure addressed the underlying disease, and therefore there is no reoccurrence or flail toe (**Figs. 20** and **21**).

Complications

Patients may experience prolonged swelling, which can be unattractive, especially for women. Recurrent painful lesion and deformity of the digits such as flail toe, misalignment, and loss of digital purchase can also be seen and may require additional surgery.[33,39–41,43,44]

Summary

Correction of the fifth digit deformity for a foot and ankle surgeon can be rewarding as well as challenging. Immense care should be taken when performing any digital procedure, especially of the fifth digits, to avoid and minimize complication rates and mainly to prevent neurovascular damage.

REFERENCES

1. Bertrand T, Selene GP. Bunionette deformity: etiology, nonsurgical management, and lateral exostectomy. Foot Ankle Clin 2011;16:679–88.
2. Ishikawa SN, Murphy GA. Lesser toe abnormalities. In: Canale ST, editor. Campbell's operative orthopaedics. 10th edition. Philadelphia, PA: Mosby; 2003. p. 4652–60.

3. Coughlin MJ. Treatment of bunionette deformity with longitudinal diaphyseal osteotomy with distal soft tissue repair. Foot Ankle 1991;11:195.
4. Ajis A, Koti M, Maffulli N, et al. Taylor's bunion: a review. J Foot Ankle Surg 2005; 44:236–45.
5. Wexler D, Grosser DM, Kile TA. Bunion and bunionette. In: Frontera WR, Silver JK, editors. Essentials of Physical Medicine and Rehabilitation. 2nd edition. Philadelphia, PA: Saunders Elsevier; 2008;chap 76.
6. Roukis TS. The tailor's bunionette deformity: a field guide to surgical correction. Clin Podiatr Med Surg 2005;22:223–45.
7. Roukis TS. Minimum-incision metatarsal osteotomies. Clin Podiatr Med Surg 2008;25:587–607.
8. Roukis TS. Central metatarsal head-neck osteotomies: indications and operative techniques. Clin Podiatr Med Surg 2005;22:197–222.
9. Haskell A, Mann RA. Foot and ankle. Biomechanics. In: DeLee JC, Drez D Jr, Miller MD, editors. DeLee & Drez's orthopaedic sports medicine, vol. 2, 3rd edition. Philadelphia: Saunders/Elsevier; 2010. p. 1865–73.
10. Baumhauer JF, Benedict FD. Osteotomies of the fifth metatarsal. Foot Ankle Clin 2001;6:3.
11. Hansen ST. Functional reconstruction of the foot and ankle. 1st edition. Philadelphia: Lippincott Williams & Wilkins; 2000. p. 264.
12. Good J, Fiala K. Digital surgery: current trends and techniques. Clin Podiatr Med Surg 2010;27:583–99.
13. Caselli MA, George DH. Foot deformities: biomechanical and pathomechanical changes associated with aging, part I. Clin Podiatr Med Surg 2003;20: 487–509.
14. Fallat L, Buckholz J. An analysis of the tailors bunion by radiographic and anatomic display. J Am Podiatry Assoc 1980;70:597.
15. Casteel CA, Sikorski A, De Yoe BE. Surgery of the central rays. Clin Podiatr Med Surg 2010;27:509–22.
16. Pontious J, Lane GD, Moritz JC, et al. Lesser metatarsal V-osteotomy for chronic intractable plantar keratosis: retrospective analysis of 40 procedures. J Am Podiatr Med Assoc 1998;88:323–31.
17. Thomas JL, Blitch EL 4th, Chaney DM, et al. Diagnosis and treatment of forefoot disorders. Section 1: digital deformities. J Foot Ankle Surg 2009;48(2):230–72.
18. Kitaoka HB, Holiday AD. Lateral condylar resection for bunionette. Clin Orthop 1992;278:183–92.
19. Dorris MF, Mandel LM. Fifth metatarsal head resection for correction of tailor's bunions and sub-fifth metatarsal head keratoma: a retrospective analysis. J Foot Surg 1991;30(3):269–75.
20. Addante JB, Chin M, Makower BL, et al. Surgical correction of tailor's bunion with resection of fifth metatarsal head and Silastic sphere implant: an 8-year follow-up study. J Foot Surg 1986;25(4):315–20.
21. Weil L, Weil LS. Osteotomies for bunionette deformity. Foot Ankle Clin 2011;16: 689–712.
22. Schuh R, Trnka HJ. Metatarsalgia: distal metatarsal osteotomies. Foot Ankle Clin 2011;16:583–95.
23. Helal B. Metatarsal osteotomy for metatarsalgia. J Bone Joint Surg Br 1975;57: 187–92.
24. Vienne P, Oesselmann M, Espinosa N, et al. Modified Coughlin procedure for surgical treatment of symptomatic tailor's bunion: a prospective follow-up study of 33 consecutive operations. Foot Ankle Int 2006;27:573–80.

25. Castle JE, Cohen AH, Docks G. Fifth metatarsal distal oblique wedge osteotomy utilizing cortical screw fixation. J Foot Surg 1992;31:478–85.
26. Gerbert J, Sgarlato TE, Subotnick SI. Preliminary study of a closing wedge osteotomy of the fifth metatarsal for correction of a tailor's bunion deformity. J Am Podiatr Assoc 1972;62(6):212–8.
27. Diebold PF, Bejjani FJ. Basal osteotomy of the fifth metatarsal with intermetatarsal pinning: a new approach to the tailor's bunion. Foot Ankle 1987;8(1):40–5.
28. LaVelle DG. Delayed union and nonunion of fractures. In: Canale ST, editor. Campbell's Operative Orthopedics. 10th edition. Vol. 3. Philadelphia, PA: Mosby; 2003. p. 3125–65.
29. Dolce M, Adamov DJ. Postoperative complication in podiatric surgery. In: Levy LA, Hetherington VJ, editors. Principles and practice of podiatric medicine, vol. 51. Brooklandville (MD): Data Trace; 2006. p. 1–14.
30. Bellacosa RA, Pollak RA. Complications of lesser metatarsal surgery. Clin Podiatr Med Surg 1991;8(2):383–97.
31. Coughlin MJ. Bunionettes. In: Coughlin MJ, Mann RA, Saltzman CL, editors. Surgery of the foot and ankle. 8th edition. Philadelphia: Mosby-Elsevier; 2007. p. 491–530.
32. McGlamry ED, Jimenez AL, Green DR. Part 1: deformities of the intermediate digits and the metatarsophalangeal joint. In: Banks AS, Downey MS, Martin DE, et al, editors. McGlamry's comprehensive textbook of foot and ankle surgery. Philadelphia: Lippincott, Williams & Wilkins; 2001. p. 253–304.
33. Mandracchia VJ, Mandi DM, Haverstock BD, et al. Lesser metatarsal and digital surgery. In: Levy LA, Hetherington VJ, editors. Principles and practice of podiatric medicine, vol. 41. Brooklandville (MD): Data Trace; 2006. p. 1–46.
34. Harmonson JK, Harkless LB. Operative procedures for the correction of hammertoe, claw toe, and mallet toe: a literature review. Clin Podiatr Med Surg 1996;13(2):211–20.
35. Coughlin MJ. Lesser toe deformities. In: Coughlin MJ, Mann RA, Saltzman CL, editors. Surgery of the foot and ankle. Philadelphia: Mosby; 2007. p. 363–464.
36. Green DR, Brekke M. Anatomy, biomechanics, and pathomechanics of lesser digital deformities. Clin Podiatr Med Surg 1996;13(2):179–200.
37. Spencer SA. Pathomechanics of common foot pathologies. In: Levy LA, Hetherington VJ, editors. Principles and practice of podiatric medicine, vol. 4. Brooklandville (MD): Data Trace; 2006. p. 1–10.
38. DiDomenico L. Essential insight on the tendon transfers for digital dysfunction. Podiatry Today 2010;23(4):44–55.
39. Coughlin MJ. Lesser-toe abnormalities. Instr Course Lect 2002;84(8):1445–69.
40. Smith TF, Pfeifer KD. Part 2: surgical repair of fifth digit deformities. In: Banks AS, Downey MS, Martin DE, et al, editors. McGlamry's comprehensive textbook of foot and ankle surgery. Philadelphia: Lippincott, Williams & Wilkins; 2001. p. 305–21.
41. Strash WW. Arthroplasty for fifth toe deformity. Clin Podiatr Med Surg 2000;27: 625–8.
42. Marek L, Giacopelli J, Granoff D. Syndactylization for the treatment of fifth toe deformities. J Am Podiatry Assoc 1991;81(5):248–52.
43. Weil L, Schilling RA. How to handle complications of hammertoe surgery. Podiatry Today 2005;18(9):1–5.
44. Coughlin MJ, Dorris J, Polk E. Operative repair of the fixed hammertoe deformity. Foot Ankle Int 2000;21(2):94–104.

New Techniques and Alternative Fixation for the Lapidus Arthrodesis

Nathan J. Young, DPM, AACFAS, AAFAS[a,b],
Charles M. Zelen, DPM, FACFAS, FACFAOM[a,b],*

KEYWORDS

- Lapidus procedure • First metatarsocuneiform arthrodesis
- Polyaxial and monoaxial locking plates • Mini TightRope • External fixation
- Arthroscopy

KEY POINTS

- Arthrodesis of the first metatarsocuneiform joint is a powerful procedure to be used in the correction of various pathologic conditions of the first ray.
- Because of its history of high rates of nonunion, many surgeons are reluctant to perform this procedure.
- Newer devices, especially the advent of locking plate technology slightly more than a decade ago, have allowed surgeons to confidently fixate the joint and help reconstruct the first ray with a lower rate of nonunion.
- Other innovative techniques and technology, such as arthroscopic fusion of the joint and the use of exceptionally strong sutures to decrease and fixate the intermetatarsal space, are still in their infancy; their long-term results remain to be seen.

INTRODUCTION

Fusion of the first metatarsocuneiform (MTC) joint was first described by Albrecht in 1911[1] but was popularized by Lapidus[2] in 1934. In his report, Lapidus described fixation of the fusion using a number zero chromic catgut suture and allowed immediate postoperative ambulation in a leather-soled shoe.[2] He abandoned the procedure for a time because of the lack of adequate internal fixation.[3] Since Lapidus' time, numerous fixation methods have been advocated, including staples, Kirschner wires (k wires), lag screws, plates, and, more recently, external fixation or locking plates.[4]

[a] Foot and Ankle Associates of Southwest Virginia, 1802 Braeburn Drive, Suite M120, Salem, VA 24153, USA; [b] Professional Education and Research Institute, 222 Walnut Avenue, Roanoke, VA 24016, USA
* Corresponding author. Foot and Ankle Associates of Southwest Virginia, 1802 Braeburn Drive, Suite M120, Salem, VA 24153, USA.
E-mail address: cmzelen@periedu.com

Clin Podiatr Med Surg 30 (2013) 423–434
http://dx.doi.org/10.1016/j.cpm.2013.04.007
0891-8422/13/$ – see front matter © 2013 Published by Elsevier Inc.
podiatric.theclinics.com

Regardless of the fixation method, one of the potential complications when performing this procedure is nonunion of the arthrodesis.[5] Before advancements in rigid internal fixation, nonunion rates for the Lapidus procedure approached 25%.[6] As a result, many surgeons were hesitant to perform the procedure.[7] After advancements in screw technology, published data suggested the nonunion rate to be between 3.3% and 12.0%.[4,8,9] Patel and colleagues[9] found the nonunion rate of the Lapidus procedure to be 5.3% in 227 feet retrospectively analyzed. Interestingly, in a systematic review of the literature, Donnenwerth and colleagues[5] evaluated published research of nearly 600 feet that had first MTC joint curettage with 2 crossed compression screws and also found the nonunion rate to be 5.3%.

Some surgeons have limited their use of the Lapidus procedure because of the risk of nonunion. Blitz[6] argues that nonunions exist even in the best hands and therefore, they should not be considered a complication but rather "an expected outcome in a low percentage of cases."[6] The Lapidus, however, remains one of the most powerful procedures in the correction of common foot pathologies, including metatarsus primus varus associated with hallux abducto valgus (HAV), first ray hypermobility, arthrosis of the first MTC joint, recurrent HAV, stabilization of the medial column, a long first metatarsal, and HAV associated with ligamentous laxity.[4,8,10,11]

In his report, Lapidus[2] described fixation of the fusion using a number zero chromic catgut suture and allowed immediate postoperative ambulation in a leather-soled shoe. He abandoned the procedure for a time because of the lack of adequate internal fixation.[3] Modern principles of bone fixation developed in 1958 by the Swiss association Arbeitsgemeinschaft fuer Osteosynthesisfragen, or AO, have improved the success rate and include anatomic reduction, rigid internal fixation, atraumatic technique on the soft tissues and bone, and early pain-free range of motion. With the advent of AO fixation, biomechanical studies have shown that the stainless steel screws are 4 times stronger and are 12 times more stable than suture fixation.[12] As such, suture or wire fixation of the Lapidus arthrodesis is no longer considered.

Although suture fixation may have been abandoned as a technique for fixation of the fusion, it still may be considered to maintain and reduce the intermetatarsal angle during a Lapidus. Arthrex offers the Mini TightRope (Arthrex, Naples, FL), which is a No. 2 FiberWire suture with 2 stainless steel buttons. This suture is a novel way to help correct the intermetatarsal angle. The Mini TightRope device is to be used as an adjunct fixation device in the Lapidus procedure. There have been several case studies by foot and ankle surgeons describing this use. Hasselman and colleagues[13] has submitted the results of this procedure for publication in 40 patients. He experienced no nonunions or malunions, no recurrence of the deformity, and he reports that the correction from the procedure is not lost over time. His technique inserts the Mini TightRope proximally through the base of the first metatarsal and into the base of the second metatarsal. This placement holds the correction during the application of the plate and screw. The Mini TightRope can also be inserted distally in the neck of the first metatarsal and secured to the second metatarsal to correct and maintain the transverse plane stability and to augment the correction of the plate and screws. Potential disadvantages may include delayed or nonunion of the fusion caused by increased tension on the medial aspect of the arthrodesis, fracture of the second metatarsal, and hallux varus. These complications can lead to significant added expense. Therefore, more studies evaluating the long-term results are needed to determine the true long-term efficacy of this type of fixation.

For many years, the gold standard in fixation of the Lapidus was by placing 2 crossing screws through the first MTC joint as made popular by Sangeorzan and Hansen[14] in 1989. Some investigators prefer the insertion of an additional screw through the first metatarsal and into the intermediate cuneiform and/or from the medial cuneiform into the intermediate cuneiform. Biomechanical research has yielded controversial results. Gruber and colleagues[8] found that crossing screws alone were equivalent in terms of rigidity compared with crossing screws with a dorsomedial plate. Cohen and colleagues[15] also found that crossing screws were stronger and provided increased rigidity when compared with a dorsal H-plate without any interfragmentary screws.[15] Klos and colleagues,[16] however, performed a biomechanical study and found that a dorsomedial locking plate with an adjunct compression screw was, in fact, superior to crossing screws. Clinically, plating with a single screw or crossing screws seems to offer superior results with increased rates of fusion and/or earlier return to weight bearing when compared with crossing screws alone.[4,7,11,17,18] Some investigators recommend plantar interfragmentary lag screw insertion combined with plating systems. This technique provides compression across the tension side of the joint.[10,11] Research has yielded good results thus far; however, it is technically more demanding and more time consuming.

Because of the notoriously high rate of complications including nonunion following the Lapidus procedures, innovators have designed plates specifically for this purpose. Newer-generation plating devices seek to provide excellent conformity to the local anatomy; allow for ease of placement of locking and nonlocking screws; provide rigidity and stability; and, in some instances, provide compression. Over the last few years, it has become more commonplace for foot and ankle surgeon to use locking plates for the Lapidus procedure primarily.[19] Examples of newer-generation Lapidus plates include the VariAx plate (Stryker, Mahwah, NJ); CP Anchorage plate (Stryker, Mahwah, NJ) (**Figs. 1** and **2**); Contours LPS (Orthofix, Lewisville, TX); FPS Lapidus plate (Osteomed, Addison, TX); Ascension Orthopedics Lapidus plate (Ascension Orthopedics, Austin, TX); Arthrex Lapidus plate (Arthrex, Naples, FL); Darco LPS plate (Wright Medical Technology, Inc, Arlington, TN); Aptus plate (Medartis, Basel, Switzerland) (**Fig. 3**); Depuy Alps plate (Biomet, Warsaw, IN); Accumed Forefoot locking plate (Acumed, Hillsboro, OR) (**Fig. 4**); and the Synthes First TMT fusion plate (Synthes, West Chester, PA).

Fixation via plating technology achieves stability in different ways, depending on whether the plate is locking or nonlocking. Nonlocking plates work by compressing the plate to bone causing static friction. Similarly, locking plates limit forces at the fracture or fusion site by acting as a single beam. This single-beam construct gives increased strength and stiffness when compared with its nonlocking plate counterparts. Because the construct acts as a single unit, it requires very high forces before screw toggle or failure occurs. Because of its increased stability these types of plates provide, they should be especially considered in the high-risk fusion.[20–23]

One disadvantage of earlier-generation locking plate systems was that they were fixed-angle, or monoaxial, systems. Occasionally, this led to difficulty during screw insertion because of the blocking of the lag screw or other hardware. In addition, with the unique contour of the first MTC joint, screws could also be placed in a less-than-optimal position because you are constrained to only one angle for insertion. Many newer-generation locking plate systems are polyaxial, which gives the surgeon the possibility to insert the screws at a different angle, thus allowing increased freedom anywhere from 10° to 15° from the center of the screw hole in any direction. Most polyaxial locking plates have holes that can accept either a locking or a nonlocking screw. The usage of a nonlocking screw in the hybrid plate provides better conformity of the plate against the bone because this nonlocking construct is able to bring the plate and the bone into close apposition. Using a mixture of nonlocking and locking screws also maintains a lower overall cost.

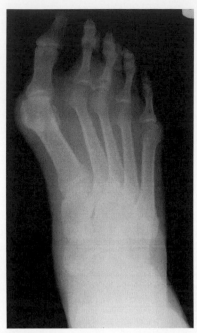

Fig. 1. Preoperative radiographs of severe bunion deformity as well as second hammertoe and elongated partially dislocated second metatarsophalangeal joint. Postoperative radiographs of the Anchorage CP plate with excellent fusion of the first metatarsal cuneiform joint, reduction of the bunion deformity, and correction of the hammertoe and second metatarsal phalangeal joint pathology.

The use of external fixation in Lapidus procedures is also a viable option. External fixation offers the ability to bear weight immediately after surgery; there is no retained internal hardware when the fixator is removed; and, when performed correctly, a predictable fusion is usually obtained.[24] A powerful indication for external fixation is in the case of revision Lapidus fusion because of infected hardware or osteomyelitis to provide an effective means for septic fusion.

Wang and Riley[24] presented 102 patients who had a Lapidus procedure with external fixation. They found that the average time to unassisted full weight bearing was 13.1 days; the average time to fusion was 5.3 weeks, with removal of the fixator at 5.5 weeks postoperatively. They had no incidences of delayed union or nonunion. They had one case of pin track irritation/infection, which resolved with appropriate pin care and antibiotics.[24] Although this study provided a complication and healing rate that is rather unparalleled in the literature, Treadwell's[25] series provided a more realistic rate of complications often seen with external fixation–related midfoot fusions. Treadwell[25] evaluated a series of 16 proximal metatarsal procedures using a rail external fixator, 11 of which were Lapidus procedures and 5 of which were base wedge osteotomies. He reported significant complications, including 10 out of 16 pin tract infections, 5 which required isolated pin removal and another 2 required removal of the entire frame because of the severity of infection. Seven patients developed hardware loosening. Two patients required long-term intravenous antibiotic therapy. Two of the 11 Lapidus procedures went on to nonunion.[25] However, Van Gompel and Dei[26] warned that it is difficult to make any conclusive statements

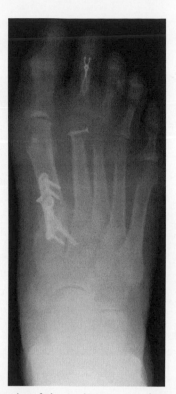

Fig. 2. Postoperative radiographs of the Anchorage CP plate with excellent fusion of the first metatarsal cuneiform joint, reduction of the bunion deformity, and correction of the hammertoe and elongated second metatarsal. Postoperative radiographs of the Anchorage CP plate with excellent fusion of the first metatarsal cuneiform joint, reduction of the bunion deformity, and correction of the hammertoe and second metatarsal phalangeal joint pathology.

about the use of external fixation in the Lapidus procedure and recommended further study with larger patient populations.

Another possible technique for Lapidus arthrodesis in the foot and ankle surgeon's armamentarium is the arthroscopic Lapidus. The arthroscopic technique may allow better visualization of the plantar and lateral side of the joint. It may allow easier and more thorough removal of the articular cartilage without needing to take the subchondral bone, which may help eliminate excessive shortening of the first ray. It may also provide better cosmesis and less scar formation, less postoperative wound pain, and less risk of infection.[27]

Lui and colleagues[28] described their technique for primary arthrodesis of the first MTC joint in *Arthroscopy* in 2005. The instrumentation that they recommend is a 2.7-mm, 30° arthroscope, a small periosteal elevator, an arthroscopic osteotome, and an arthroscopic awl. A 21-gauge needle is inserted into the joint and it is inflated with 2 to 3 mL of sterile normal saline. Two arthroscopy ports are then made plantar medially and dorsomedial to the joint. After visualization of the joint using the arthroscope, the articular cartilage is denuded using the osteotome and periosteal elevator leaving the subchondral bone intact. Arthroscopic awls are then used to perform microfracture to the subchondral bone. After reduction of the intermetatarsal angle and with some mild plantar flexion, a 4.0-mm cannulated screw is inserted in a

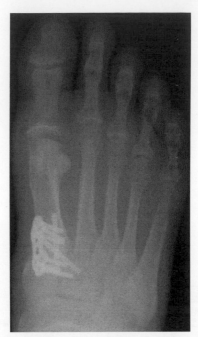

Fig. 3. Polyaxial locking plate used here for neutralization allows for angular insertion of the screws based on position surgeon assesses as most appropriate. Herbert headless screws are used for joint compression and metatarsal-intercuneiform stability.

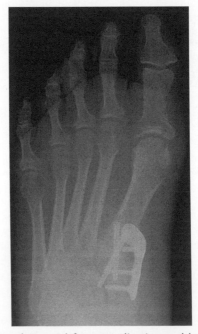

Fig. 4. Mono axial locking plate used for neutralization and headless Herbert screws for joint compression. Also note the Akin osteotomy fixated with resorbable screw fixation.

lag-screw fashion from proximal dorsal to distal plantar to compress the joint. A second 4.0-mm positioning screw is inserted from the base of the first metatarsal to the base of the second metatarsal, which is subsequently removed at 12 weeks. Patients are kept non–weight bearing for an extended period of time, up to 12 weeks with this procedure. Arthroscopy of the first MTC joint may provide an effective minimally invasive means of the Lapidus procedure.

Lui and colleagues and Lui[27,28] reported single case studies of the arthroscopic technique. They described a case of primary arthrodesis using arthroscopy and also a case of revision arthrodesis using arthroscopy. Michels and colleagues[29] performed arthroscopic Lapidus fusion on 5 patients and reported that the hallux valgus angle improved by 25.6°, the intermetatarsal angle improved by 10.6°, and shortening of the first ray was limited to 2.7 mm. They had fusion in all 5 patients. Lui and colleagues[28] recommend that this technique only be used by surgeons who are familiar with small joint arthroscopy because of the high degree of technical demand.

Bone healing across a fracture or an osteotomy typically takes 6 to 8 weeks to achieve in a healthy individual. Because the Lapidus procedure has a high risk of nonunions, many surgeons will limit their patients to a strict non–weight-bearing protocol during this time period.[5] Prolonged non–weight bearing can have deleterious effects for patients, such as disuse osteopenia, muscle atrophy, weight gain, deep vein thrombosis, and pulmonary embolism.[30] After periods of prolonged non–weight bearing, it is vital to gradually increase patients' weight-bearing activities to prevent injury secondary to the bone and muscle atrophy. It is also essential to provide proper prophylaxis with an anticoagulant during the early non–weight-bearing period to help prevent deep vein thrombosis and pulmonary embolism.

Because of the disadvantages of prolonged non–weight bearing, there is a growing amount of research that advocates earlier weight bearing after a Lapidus fusion. Some investigators recommend weight bearing at 2 weeks postoperatively once the surgical wounds have healed.[5–7] Others recommend near-immediate weight bearing.[17] When considering early weight bearing, it is vital to consider multiple factors, including the patients' age, activity level, smoking status, usage of nonsteroidal antiinflammatory drugs, obesity, and whether they are neuropathic or not.[6] Sangeorzan and Hansen[14] promoted early weight bearing and found 92% union rate. Sorenson and colleagues[7] applied locking plates for a Lapidus fusion and allowed weight bearing at 2 weeks and had 100% union. Saxena and colleagues[11] found no difference in fusion rates between crossing screws and locking plates for Lapidus fusion but did find that the locking-plate group ambulated at 4 weeks instead of 6 weeks in the crossing-screw group. Basile and colleagues[17] allowed immediate postoperative partial weight bearing by fusing the first MTC joint with crossing screws and also inserting a stabilizing percutaneous k wire and compared the results with their control group who had crossing screws only and were non–weight bearing for 6 weeks in 41 patients. Neither group had nonunions or malunions. Although very little research exists on the definitive length of non–weight bearing after a Lapidus, existing research may indicate that with newer plating options and in selected individuals, earlier weight bearing may be appropriate.

AUTHORS' SURGICAL TECHNIQUE FOR LAPIDUS ARTHRODESIS

With the patient placed on the operating table in the supine position, a well-padded pneumatic calf tourniquet is placed on the operative extremity. If needed, an ipsilateral hip bump is placed to help adduct the extremity.

A dorsomedial skin incision is made from 1 cm proximal to the first MTC joint and extended to the level of the hallux interphalangeal joint. Attention is first directed to the metatarsal head. The medial eminence is resected and a lateral release is performed if indicated. Next, with attention directed proximally, a longitudinal incision is made at the first MTC joint to expose the joint. Next, the first MTC joint surfaces are carefully resected with a triangular cut made on the cuneiform with more bone taken laterally than medially to reduce the intermetatarsal angle, and a straight cut is made over the metatarsal. The medial aspect of the second metatarsal is denuded; if needed, a small section of bone is taken from the lateral aspect of the first metatarsal, which allows for lateral translation of the first metatarsal and further deformity correction. Finally, some plantar flexion of the first metatarsal is created to compensate for the shortening of the ray. Fenestrating the joint surface with a 1.5-mm drill is recommended after bone resection to obtain further bleeding channels for healing.

Once the joint surfaces are prepared and the deformity reduced, one guidewire is directed from the dorsal aspect of the base of the first metatarsal into the plantar aspect of the medial cuneiform through the MTC joint. Another guidewire is inserted from the plantar medial aspect of the base of the first metatarsal and directed proximally and laterally into the intermediate cuneiform. Headless compression screws are then inserted. Positioning is confirmed using intraoperative fluoroscopy. After insertion of the compression screws, a dorsomedial locking plate is then applied.

The wounds are closed in anatomic layers, and a dry sterile dressing is applied. A well-padded posterior splint is applied. At the 2-week follow-up, the sutures are removed and a short leg fiberglass cast is applied for an additional 4 weeks. Light weight bearing is permitted after the second week.

Case Presentation

This patient is a 21-year-old woman who presented after a recent failed Lapidus arthrodesis. She underwent surgery 3 months before and had gapping and pain at the first MTC joint. Her past medical history was significant for smoking, and her social history significant for being a single mother with a small child. The initial treating physician related she was weight bearing immediately postoperatively because of caring for her young child, which was thought to be the cause of the joint distraction. Her treating doctor offered her a bone stimulator; but because of the significant joint distraction appreciated on radiograph, she opted for surgery and was referred to the authors for revision.

On physical examination, her neurovascular status was intact and normal. She did have some swelling around the surgical site. She had specific pinpoint pain and discomfort over the first MTC joint. She otherwise had good range of motion and muscle strength. Radiographs show crossing headless compression screws and a distracted nonunion of the right first MTC joint (**Figs. 5** and **6**).

The surgery was performed removing the original hardware, and there was a clear nonunion across the joint. The joint was re-resected to good bleeding bone, and the joint surfaces were fenestrated. Headless compression screws were then used to compress the fusion site and to slightly plantar flex the first ray to accommodate the shortening from the resected bone. Vitos Bone Graft Substitute (Stryker, Mahwah, NJ) with bone marrow aspirate was inserted into the osteotomy to enhance healing. A 4.5-mm Herbert compression screw was placed to compress the joint surfaces. A polyaxial Variax H-plate (Stryker, Mahwah, NJ) was then placed. The plate provided substantial rigidity and neutralization across the fusion site (**Figs. 7** and **8**).

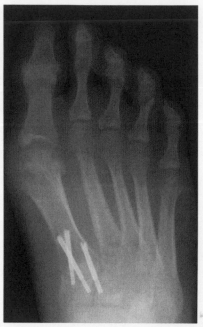

Fig. 5. Preoperative radiographs show diastasis at the first metatarsal cuneiform joint with complete nonunion.

The patient was kept non–weight bearing for a total of 6 weeks initially in a splint and then in a fiberglass cast. She was then progressed to a Controlled Ankle Motion boot (CAM boot) and was in tennis shoes at 8 weeks. At nearly 12 months postoperative, she remains very pleased with the correction of her deformity and has no pain. Radiographs reveal solid bony union at the first MTC joint (see **Figs. 7** and **8**). The original surgeon may have considered the history of smoking and her small child she had to care for; thus, had a locking plate been used primarily in this case, the early weight bearing that led to joint distraction may never have occurred.

CLINICAL RESULTS IN THE LITERATURE

Most of the recent publications regarding the Lapidus procedure seem to be directed toward locking plate technology. Clearly, locking plates offer a very stable construct that can decrease the risk of nonunions.

Locking plates provide a very rigid construct, which lends itself to good bone healing. In a series of 128 (144 feet), Wilde and colleagues[31] evaluated the Lapidus

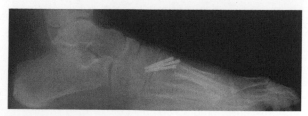

Fig. 6. Preoperative radiographs show diastasis at the first metatarsal cuneiform joint with complete nonunion.

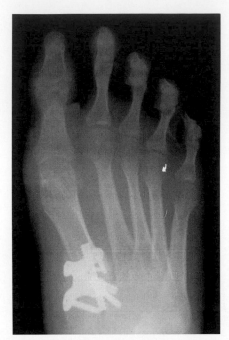

Fig. 7. A 12-month postoperative radiograph from the revision Lapidus shows good union across the joint. Note the slight plantar flexion of the first ray to accommodate for the shortening of the ray.

procedure using polyaxial locking plates and found a union rate of 98.6%. Sorensen and colleagues[7] had a 100% rate of union with interfragmentary screw and dorsomedial locking plate fixation. They also found that full weight bearing with ambulation was possible at 2 weeks postoperatively.[7] DeVries and colleagues[4] performed a Lapidus on 143 patients using either crossing screws or a dorsomedial locking plate with no interfragmentary compression. They found a union rate of 89.4% for the crossed-screw group and 98.5% for the locking-plate group. They also found that the locking plate was bearing full weight at 7.8 weeks instead of 8.8 weeks.[4] Saxena and colleagues[11] performed the Lapidus procedure on 40 patients with either crossing lag screws or a plantar lag screw with locking plate fixation. They found no significant difference in the rate of nonunions between the two groups; however, they did find that the locking-plate group was able to bear weight at 4 weeks as opposed to 6 weeks in the crossing-screw group.[11]

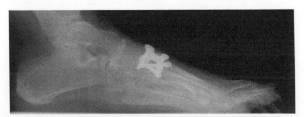

Fig. 8. A 12-month postoperative radiograph from the revision Lapidus shows good union across the joint. Note the slight plantar flexion of the first ray to accommodate for the shortening of the ray.

SUMMARY

Arthrodesis of the first MTC joint is a powerful and durable procedure to help correct moderate to severe hallux valgus and/or first ray hypermobility. However, painful nonunion remains a notoriously high potential outcome, between 3.3% and 12.0%. Although some investigators may advocate early weight bearing when using crossing lag screws and locking plates, the authors think that larger prospective and random- ized clinical research needs to be conducted to determine the length of non–weight bearing after a Lapidus procedure. Because of the costs and risks associated with revision surgery, it may be more beneficial to use locking plates with lag screws and to keep patients non–weight bearing for a minimum of at least 2 weeks. Research regarding locking plates seems very promising, and data so far show lower rates of nonunion. External fixation for Lapidus may provide excellent fixation and allow earlier weight bearing, but care for and complications of the external device may be a concern to surgeons and patients. Innovative fixation techniques, such as the Mini TightRope or arthroscopic fusion, are quite new but have very little published data supporting their use. Regardless of the fixation, proper joint preparation and good compression are fundamental in attempting to avoid a failed first MTC fusion.

REFERENCES

1. Albrecht GH. The pathology and treatment of hallux valgus (Russian). Russk Vrach 1911;10:14–9.
2. Lapidus PW. The operative correction of the metatarsus varus primus in hallux valgus. Surg Gynecol Obstet 1934;58:183–91.
3. Hansen ST Jr. Hallux valgus surgery. Morton and Lapidus were right! Clin Podiatr Med Surg 1996;13:347–54.
4. DeVries JG, Granata JD, Hyer CF. Fixation of first tarsometatarsal arthrodesis: a retrospective comparative cohort of two techniques. Foot Ankle Int 2011;32(2): 158–62.
5. Donnenwerth MP, Borkosky SL, Abicht BP, et al. Rate of nonunion after first metatarsal-cuneiform arthrodesis using joint curettage and two crossed compres- sion screw fixation: a systematic review. J Foot Ankle Surg 2011;50(6):707–9.
6. Blitz NM. Early weightbearing of the Lapidus bunionectomy: is it feasible? Clin Podiatr Med Surg 2012;29:367–81.
7. Sorensen MD, Berlet GC, Hyer CF. Results of Lapidus arthrodesis and locked plating with early weight bearing. Foot Ankle Spec 2009;2(5):227–33.
8. Gruber F, Sinkov VS, Bae SY, et al. Crossed screws versus dorsomedial locking plate with compression screws for first metatarsocuneiform arthrodesis: a cadaver study. Foot Ankle Int 2008;29(9):927–30.
9. Patel S, Ford LA, Etcheverry J, et al. Modified Lapidus arthrodesis: rate of nonunion in 227 cases. J Foot Ankle Surg 2004;43(1):37–42.
10. Cottom JM. Fixation of the Lapidus arthrodesis with a plantar interfragmentary screw and medial low profile locking plate. J Foot Ankle Surg 2012;51(4):517–22.
11. Saxena A, Nguyen A, Nelson E. Lapidus bunionectomy: early evaluation of crossed lag screws versus locking plate with plantar lag screw. J Foot Ankle Surg 2009;48(2):170–9.
12. Calder JD, Holligdale JP, Pearse MF. Screw versus suture fixation of Mitchell's osteotomy: a prospective, randomised study. J Bone Joint Surg Br 1999;81(4):621–4.
13. Hasselman CT. Success story: Lapidus plate. Mini TightRope Lapidus technique. Distal extremities orthopedic update, spring 2012. Arthrex newsletter. Accessed October 8, 2012.

14. Sangeorzan BJ, Hansen ST. Modified Lapidus procedure for hallux valgus. Foot Ankle 1989;9(6):262–6.
15. Cohen DA, Parks BG, Schon LC. Screw fixation compared to H-locking plate fixation for first metatarsocuneiform arthrodesis: a biomechanical study. Foot Ankle Int 2005;26(11):984–9.
16. Klos K, Gueorguiev B, Mückley T, et al. Stability of medial locking plate and compression screw versus two crossed screws for Lapidus arthrodesis. Foot Ankle Int 2010;31(2):158–63.
17. Basile P, Cook EA, Cook JJ. Immediate weight bearing following modified Lapidus arthrodesis. J Foot Ankle Surg 2010;49(5):459–64.
18. Scranton PE, Coetzee JC, Carreira D. Arthrodesis of the first metatarsocuneiform joint: a comparative study of fixation methods. Foot Ankle Int 2009;30(4):341–5.
19. Grassia T. "Surgeons prefer polyaxial locking plate for hallux valgus." Orthopaedics Today Europe 2011, Issue 5. Online.
20. Haidukewych GJ. Innovations in locking plate technology. J Am Acad Orthop Surg 2004;12(4):205–12.
21. Haidukewych GJ, Ricci W. Locked plating in orthopaedic trauma: a clinical update. J Am Acad Orthop Surg 2008;16(6):347–55.
22. Königshausen M, Kübler L, Godry H, et al. Clinical outcome and complications using a polyaxial locking plate in the treatment of displaced proximal humerus fractures. A reliable system? Injury 2012;43(2):223–31.
23. Voigt C, Geisler A, Hepp P, et al. Are polyaxially locked screws advantageous in the plate osteosynthesis of proximal humeral fractures in the elderly? A prospective randomized clinical observational study. J Orthop Trauma 2011;25(10):596–602.
24. Wang JC, Riley BM. A new fixation technique for the Lapidus bunionectomy. J Am Podiatr Med Assoc 2005;95(4):405–9.
25. Treadwell JR. Rail external fixation for stabilization of closing base wedge osteotomies and Lapidus procedures: a retrospective analysis of sixteen cases. J Foot Ankle Surg 2005;44(6):429–36.
26. Van Gompel JR, Dei RL. Rail external fixation for stabilization of closing base wedge osteotomies and Lapidus procedures: a retrospective analysis of sixteen cases. J Foot Ankle Surg 2006;45(3):192–3.
27. Lui TH. Symptomatic first metatarsocuneiform nonunion revised by arthroscopic Lapidus technique. J Foot Ankle Surg 2012;51(5):656–9.
28. Lui TH, Chan KB, Ng S. Arthroscopic Lapidus arthrodesis. Arthroscopy 2005;21(12):1516.e1–4.
29. Michels F, Guillo S, de Lavigne C, et al. The arthroscopic Lapidus procedure. Foot Ankle Surg 2011;17(1):25–8.
30. Kadous A, Abdelgawad AA, Kanlic E. Deep venous thrombosis and pulmonary embolism after surgical treatment of ankle fractures: a case report and review of literature. J Foot Ankle Surg 2012;51:457–63.
31. Wilde E, Schulz AP, Heinrichs G, et al. Retrospective analysis of hallux valgus therapy by Lapidus arthrodesis with polyaxial locking plates. Poster session presented at: 12th EFORT Congress 2011. Copenhagen, Denmark, June 1–4.

Advances in Forefoot Trauma

J. Randolph Clements, DPM[a],*, Robert Schopf, DPM[b]

KEYWORDS

- Jones fracture • Forefoot trauma • Metatarsal fractures • Soft tissue defects

KEY POINTS

- Multiple fixation options are available for forefoot fracture management.
- Open fracture management has improved with advances in wound management and surgical techniques.
- The use of solid screw fixation and Jones fractures is preferable.

INTRODUCTION

Trauma involving the forefoot can cause protracted recovery and prolonged disability.[1] Fractures of the metatarsals account for approximately 80% of all fractures of the foot and ankle.[2] Trauma to the first metatarsal and first metatarsal phalangeal joint create significant functional impairment because of the dynamic nature of the first ray. These injuries usually occur as a result of a high-energy mechanism. Fractures of the central metatarsals are quite common and easily treated with nonsurgical treatments or straightforward surgical management. Fractures of the fifth metatarsal are also quite common. In this article, the authors provide a historical perspective of injuries involving the forefoot and also include recent advances in the management of these injuries. Recent advances in technology, both in soft tissue management and fracture management, have allowed clinicians to improve clinical outcomes.

ANATOMY

The first metatarsal is considerably wider and stronger than the lesser metatarsals. It is thought that one-third of the body weight is transferred through the first metatarsal phalangeal joint during gait. The first metatarsal is covered in cartilage proximally and distally. The proximal aspect is reniform, or kidney-shaped, and articulates with

The authors listed above have identified no professional or financial affiliation for themselves or their spouse/partner.

[a] Surgery, Virginia Tech Carilion School of Medicine, Carilion Clinic Orthopedics, 3 Riverside Circle, Roanoke, VA 24014, USA; [b] PGY-1, Carilion Clinic Podiatric Medicine and Surgery, 3 Riverside Circle, Roanoke, VA 24014, USA

* Corresponding author.

E-mail address: jrclements@carilionclinic.org

Clin Podiatr Med Surg 30 (2013) 435–444
http://dx.doi.org/10.1016/j.cpm.2013.04.005
0891-8422/13/$ – see front matter © 2013 Elsevier Inc. All rights reserved.

the first cuneiform. The distal aspect articulates with the base of the proximal phalanx and the sesamoid complex. The distal aspect is round to allow for sagittal plane motion of the first metatarsal phalangeal joint. The sesamoid complex is held in position by the medial and lateral flexor hallucis brevis muscles. The 2 heads of the aductor hallucis attach on the lateral side of the fibular sesamoid. A portion of the abductor hallucis inserts on the medial side of the tibial sesamoid. The deep transverse intermetatarsal ligament also contributes to sesamoid stabilization and helps to maintain the sesamoid relationship to the lesser metatarsals. This unique anatomic relationship makes little displacement of the sesamoid complex intolerable.

The first metatarsal phalangeal joint has a vertical and transverse access. The vertical axis allows for abduction and adduction. The transverse axis allows for dorsiflexion and plantar flexion. During propulsion, approximately 65° of dorsiflexion is needed at the first metatarsal phalangeal joint. A reduction, either structurally or functionally, in first metatarsal phalangeal joint motion results in a condition known as hallux limitus.

MECHANISM

Injuries to the first metatarsal phalangeal joint are typically caused by direct trauma. Most of the trauma involving the first metatarsal phalangeal joint occurs from hyper dorsiflexion mechanisms.[3,4] These mechanisms can create dislocations with or without an osseous component. These injuries can be open or closed. The open wound is typically plantar due to excessive tension placed on the plantar skin tearing in a hyperextension injury. The skin defect can be dorsal if the direct force is applied to the dorsal surface.

DIAGNOSIS

Subtle injuries to the first metatarsal phalangeal joint are often difficult to diagnose initially. If the patient has a hyperextension mechanism, the clinician should maintain a high index of suspicion for an injury to the first metatarsal phalangeal joint or sesamoid complex. Higher-energy injuries make diagnosing first metatarsal phalangeal joint pathology easier because they are often associated with gross deformity. Higher-energy mechanisms include blunt trauma, lawnmower injuries, gunshot wounds, and motor vehicle accidents. These injuries often create a composite defect involving soft tissue and bone. Depending on the size of the soft tissue and osseous defect, the injury may require amputation. Alternatives to amputation are discussed later in this article.

Standard 3-plane radiographs should be used for initial assessment of the skeletal injury. Fractures and dislocations involving the first metatarsal phalangeal joint should be recognized on plain radiography. Subtle injuries to the metatarsal, phalanx, or sesamoid complex may require advanced imaging, such as bone scintigraphy, computed tomography (CT), or magnetic resonance imaging (MRI). Bone scintigraphy and MRI are very sensitive modalities. CT is most helpful in determining fracture fragment size, articular involvement, and surgical planning.

TREATMENT OF FRACTURES
Open Fractures

Open fracture management of the first metatarsal phalangeal joint should follow standard open fracture management protocols. These protocols were initially outlined by Gustilo and Anderson.[5] These should be treated with prompt irrigation and debridement, appropriate antibiotic coverage, and skeletal stabilization. If there is adequate soft tissue coverage, definitive fixation with internal constructs is indicated. If the soft tissue defect is too large, the injury should be stabilized with an external fixator. The soft tissue defect is often treated with negative-pressure devices until a definitive soft tissue coverage plan is determined.

In cases of minimal soft tissue defect and minimal degloving, a negative-pressure wound closure device and delayed split thickness skin graft can be used. If there are segmental bone defects, autogenous bone grafting is preferred.

Nondisplaced Fractures

Nondisplaced or minimally displaced phalangeal fractures are often amenable to nonsurgical treatment. These injuries are successfully treated in a short-leg cast for 4 to 6 weeks. In some cases, a removable immobilizer boot or fracture shoe is acceptable. In these cases, diligent follow-up with serial radiographs should be considered to ensure that subsequent displacement of the fragments has not occurred.

The same practice can be applied to nondisplaced or minimally displaced fractures of the first metatarsal. Sammarco and Conti[6] have recommended a non–weight bearing cast for 2 to 3 weeks followed by a walking cast for an additional 3 weeks. Others have supported earlier weight bearing.[7] Either method is acceptable; however, the clinician should transition the patient back to soft shoes very deliberately. If the patient continues to complain of discomfort, the patient should be immobilized for a longer period of time.

Central Metatarsal Fractures

The second, third, and fourth metatarsals are considered the central metatarsals. In this article, the first and fifth metatarsals are addressed separately because of the complexity of management. Stress fractures of the central metatarsals are common and are covered in a later subsection.

The central metatarsals consist of a head, neck, shaft, and base. The head of the metatarsal articulates with the base of the proximal phalanx. The neck is the junction of the epiphysis and the diaphysis. The diaphyseal (shaft) segment is the largest segment of the metatarsal. The second and third metatarsals articulate with the second and third cuneiform, respectively. The fourth metatarsal articulates with the medial half of the cuboid.

Treatment

There are a variety of fracture patterns that affect the central metatarsals. It is important to consider the location and fracture patterns when deciding the most appropriate treatment. Most fractures involving the metatarsal head or neck should be treated nonsurgically; however, sagittal split metatarsal head fractures need open reduction with internal fixation. Other fractures of the metatarsal head and neck are more forgiving and afford the clinician the option of nonsurgical management. The plane of deformity is paramount in making this decision. Patients with significant transverse plane deformity can have satisfactory results with nonsurgical care. However, sagittal plane displacement is less acceptable. Rockwood and Green report greater than 3 to 4 mm of displacement in the sagittal plane should be treated operatively.[8,9] Sagittal plane deformity should treated aggressively to avoid painful plantar keratosis.

Fractures of the metatarsal shaft can also be treated nonsurgically. If the fracture is relatively nondisplaced, short-leg casting or removable cast boot are appropriate.[1] When the fracture is displaced and surgical treatment is being considered, the pattern of the fracture helps determine the most appropriate fixation. A vertically oriented fracture can be treated in with a 0.062-inch or 0.045-inch retrograde Kirschner wire

(K-wire).[10] Spiral fractures would be most appropriately stabilized with interfragmentary fixation. The placement of this screw is challenging because of the adjacent metatarsals interfering with the surgeon's ability to place the screw at the correct angle. Because of this, dorsal plating is recommended. This construct serves as a neutralization plating construct and simply maintains bone position until the bone has healed. High-energy mechanisms often result in comminuted metatarsal shaft fractures. Bridge plating works well in this application. Bridge plating concepts allow the surgeon to stabilize the fracture both proximally and distally while bridging or spanning the area of central comminution. This provides stabilization of the fracture without disrupting the biology around the fracture. Another option for stabilizing these fractures is external fixation (**Fig. 1**). This technique is most useful in highly comminuted or open fractures. The surgeon should pay close attention to the metatarsal declination angle when using external fixation. The external fixation bars should be oriented parallel to the long axis of the metatarsal, thus will prevent sagittal plane malalignment and malunion or nonunion of the metatarsal.

Open fractures of the metatarsals rarely result in large segmental bone defects. The same is true with the soft tissue; however, high-energy mechanisms (ie, gunshot wounds or lawnmower injuries) will have large soft tissue defects. Most of these injuries can be treated with irrigation and debridement, primary wound closure, negative-pressure wound-closure devices, and skin grafting. Composite defects consist of both bone and soft tissue defects. These create an enormous challenge to the surgeon (**Figs. 2** and **3**). Options for treatment include bone grafting and free tissue transfer or osteocutaneous free flap coverage (**Figs. 4** and **5**).[11]

Stress fractures of the central metatarsals

Stress fractures rarely occur due to acute trauma. In most cases, the patients have an underlying foot deformity that is aggravated by recurrent and repetitive activity. Other underlying biologic issues should be considered as prodromal. These include osteoporosis, vitamin D deficiency, menopause, and obesity. Patients with forefoot pain and stress fracture should also be evaluated for equinus. A tight heel cord can increase the forefoot pressures, resulting in stress fracture. This concept is often overlooked as a cause of metatarsal stress fractures.

Most stress fractures can be treated nonoperatively. Typically 4 to 6 weeks in an orthopedic walking boot is sufficient and in a rare instance surgery may be needed if nonoperative treatment fails to heal the fracture.

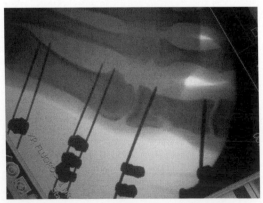

Fig. 1. Definitive fixation of open proximal phalanx fracture using mini external fixator.

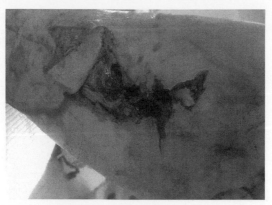

Fig. 2. Dorsal wound from shotgun wound to foot.

Fifth Metatarsal Fractures

Fractures of the fifth metatarsal are common injuries. Studies have shown that up to 75% of all metatarsal fractures occur in the fifth metatarsal. Most of these fractures involve the base of the fifth metatarsal, but a variety of distal fifth metatarsal fractures involving the head, neck, and diaphysis are seen with regularity. Like most fractures, the decision to treat these operatively or nonoperatively depends on the fracture location, angular deformity, and displacement. Sagittal plane position of the distal fragment should be carefully scrutinized on the lateral radiograph. A moderate amount of transverse plane angulation of the distal fragment is acceptable, but significant sagittal plane displacement is more problematic if not reduced. Fracture involving the base of the fifth metatarsal should be given careful consideration because of its paucity of vascular supply. Operative management in these fractures may be performed without having significant deformity or displacement.

Biologic anatomy of the fifth metatarsal

Jaworek[12] first investigated the intrinsic vascular supply of the fifth metatarsal. The primary nutrient artery of the fifth metatarsal enters at the diaphyseal of the bone. This

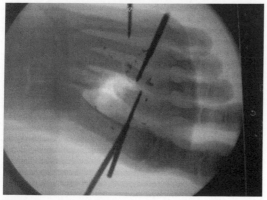

Fig. 3. A-P radiograph of gun shot wound to foot demonstrates segmental bone loss in 2nd metatarsal.

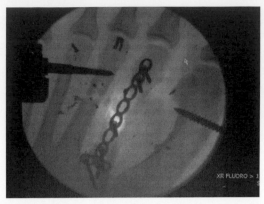

Fig. 4. Post free osteocutaneous free flap reconstruction. Bone void filled with free tissue transfer from distal radius. The bone and graft are stabilized using a bridge plating technique.

nutrient artery forms a plexus of small vessels that anastomose vascularity to the metaphyseal portion of the bone. This leads the metaphyseal portion well supplied, whereas the diaphyseal cortical bone is less vascularized. The deplete vascularity of the fifth metatarsal has been implicated as the cause for the increased incidence of delayed and nonunion in proximal diaphyseal fractures. It is also postulated that the poor prognosis of bone healing is due to the transverse fracture line in the area of the proximal diaphyseal. It is thought that this fracture line in fracture orientation disrupts the nutrient artery as it enters the cortex (**Fig. 6**).

Distal fifth metatarsal fractures

Isolated fractures of the metatarsal head are rare injuries and usually occur secondary to a direct trauma. These injuries are usually treated conservatively unless significant sagittal displacement of the head is present. The patient is typically immobilized in a below-knee cast or fracture boot for 4 to 6 weeks. If the fracture fails to unite or subsequently displaces enough to become symptomatic, a resection of the fifth metatarsal head can be considered. However, this is not suggested as a primary treatment. Fine-wire fixation or, in more severe deformity, dorsal or dorsal lateral plating may be considered if operative treatment is needed.

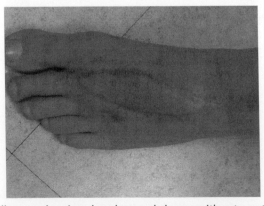

Fig. 5. 6 Month follow up showing dorsal wound closure with osteocutaneous free flap.

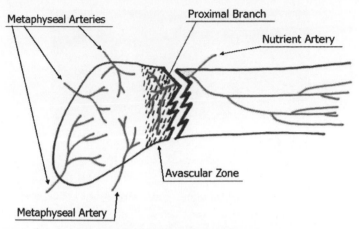

Fig. 6. Diagram showing blood supply to 5th metatarsal.

Diaphyseal fractures of the fifth metatarsal

Diaphyseal fractures of the fifth metatarsal are usually short oblique, proximal-dorsal to distal-plantar, in orientation. This fracture is commonly referred to as a dancer's fracture. The fracture occurs as a result of ground reactive forces acting distally against a stable proximal metatarsal base.

They often are associated with a moderate degree of displacement and shortening because of the obliquity of the fracture. This fracture pattern is more unstable than transverse fractures in the same location. Conservative treatment with short-leg casting may be considered if the fracture is well aligned. Open reduction with internal fixation may also be accomplished with the use of small cortical screws or small plating systems.

Comminuted fractures of the fifth metatarsal may not respond well to nonsurgical treatment. In the presence of heavy comminution, achieving mechanical stability of the fracture is often difficult. In these cases, bridge plating works well. There are also plating systems available that offer more versatile screw orientation. These are very useful in situations of comminution. Also, use of external fixation should be considered when these fractures are not amenable to internal fixation.

Proximal fractures of the fifth metatarsal

Fractures of the proximal diaphyseal portion of the fifth metatarsal are often referred to as Jones fractures. These are typically caused by an inversion force creating an avulsion at the base of the fifth metatarsal. A true Jones fracture is an acute fracture at the proximal end of the shaft near the metadiaphyseal junction.[13] If the fracture is treated nonoperatively, reports show up to 72% to 93% chance of healing. It is important to note that these fractures should be nondisplaced if conservative treatment is chosen. Nondisplaced fractures that are treated nonoperatively should be treated for 6 weeks in a non–weight-bearing short-leg cast with gradual transition to weight bearing in an orthopedic walking boot.

For acute displaced fractures of the fifth metatarsal, surgical treatment should be considered. Traditionally, surgical treatment had been reserved for high-performance athletes[14]; however, all patients with any displacement of their Jones fracture should be considered for surgical management. Intramedullary screw fixation is often recommended. Cannulated screws can be used but do not offer equivocal strength to solid screws. Cannulated screws are much less technically demanding.

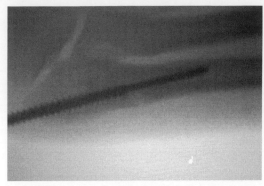

Fig. 7. Demonstrates tapping over cannulated guide wire prior to screw placement.

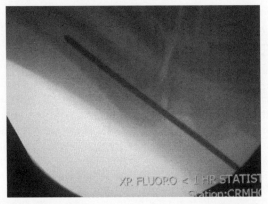

Fig. 8. Placement of cannulated guide wire into 5th metatarsal base fracture.

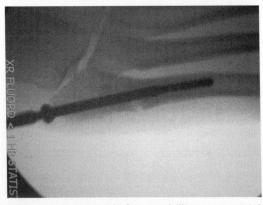

Fig. 9. Cannulated guide wire is removed after, predrilling, countersinking, and measuring are complete.

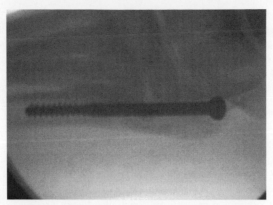

Fig. 10. Solid screw is placed after using cannulated instrumentation.

The authors recommend using cannulated instrumentation but inserting a solid screw (**Fig. 7**). This is generally achieved by using a standard cannulated guidewire followed by the appropriate cannulated drill bit. After countersinking and measuring, the cannulated guidewire is removed and the appropriate-size solid screw is inserted. Because there are minimal discrepancies in drill bit size and outer diameter of the screw, this technique allows the surgeon to use cannulated instrumentation when inserting a solid screw. No statistically significant differences have been reported between titanium and stainless steel.[15]

Other adjuncts have been suggested to improve the patient's outcome. In addition to open reduction and internal fixation, external bone stimulation has been suggested. There are multiple external bone stimulator options that are available. These devices work by low-intensity pulsed ultrasound, capacitated coupling, and pulsed electromagnetic field.

Additionally, the use of autogenous bone grafting at the time of surgery has been shown to improve outcomes.[16]

Smaller avulsion fractures can be treated with tension band wiring. When fracture fragments are too small to accommodate a standard screw, the tension band technique is the best option. The tension band technique is achieved by placing 2 parallel K-wires through the avulsion fracture. Next, a pilot hole is drilled in the diaphysis of the fifth metatarsal. An 18-gauge or 20-gauge surgical wire is then used to provide compression and neutralization to the fracture (**Figs. 8–10**). The use of 3 small wires to fixate a fifth metatarsal fracture has also been described.[17] This technique allows for a more minimally invasive approach while still providing adequate stabilization. If this technique is used, the surgeon should be conscious of the orientation of the wires. The wires should be in multiple planes to optimize neutralization.

REFERENCES

1. Morrissey E. Metatarsal fractures. J Bone Joint Surg Am 1946;28:594–602.
2. The Podiatry Institute, editor. McGlamry's comprehensive textbook of foot and ankle surgery. Philadelphia, PA: Lippincott Williams & Wilkins; 2012.
3. Brunet JA. Pathomechanics of complex dislocation of the first metatarsophalangeal joint. Clin Orthop 1996;332:126–31.
4. Jahss MH. Traumatic dislocation of the first metatarsophalangeal joint. Foot Ankle 1980;1:15–21.

5. Gustilo RB, Anderson JT. Prevention of infection in the treatment of one thousand and twenty-five open fractures of long bones: retrospective and prospective analyses. J Bone Joint Surg Am 1976;58:453–8.

6. Sammarco GJ, Conti SF. Surgical treatment of neuroarthropathic foot deformity. Foot Ankle Int 1998;19:102–9.

7. Mann RA, Coughlin MJ, editors. Surgery of the foot. Philadelphia, PA: C.V. Mosby; 1993.

8. Bucholz RW, Heckman JD, Court-Brown CM, et al, editors. Rockwood and Green's fractures in adults: two volumes plus integrated content website. Philadelphia, PA: Lippincott Williams & Wilkins; 2009.

9. Schenck RC Jr, Heckman JD. Fractures and dislocations of the forefoot: operative and nonoperative management. J Am Acad Orthop Surg 1995;3:70–8.

10. Kim HN, Park YJ, Kim GL, et al. Closed antegrade intramedullary pinning for reduction and fixation of metatarsal fractures. J Foot Ankle Surg 2012;51:445–9.

11. Clements JR, Miersch C, Bravo CJ. Management of combined soft tissue and osseous defect of the midfoot with a free osteocutaneous radial forearm flap: a case report. J Foot Ankle Surg 2012;51:118–22.

12. Jaworek TE. The intrinsic vascular supply to the first and lesser metatarsal. Surgical considerations. Sixth annual Northlake Surgical Seminar. Chicago, 1976.

13. Jones R. Fracture of the base of the fifth metatarsal bone by indirect violence. Ann Surg 1902;35:697–700.

14. Hens J, Mortens M. Surgical treatment of Jones fractures. Arch Orthop Trauma Surg 1990;109:277–9.

15. DeVries JG, Cuttica DJ, Hyer CF. Cannulated screw fixation of Jones fifth metatarsal fractures: a comparison of titanium and stainless steel screw fixation. J Foot Ankle Surg 2011;50:207–12.

16. Tsukada S, Ikeda H, Seki Y, et al. Intramedullary screw fixation with bone autografting to treat proximal fifth metatarsal metaphyseal-diaphyseal fracture in athletes: a case series. Sports Med Arthrosc Rehabil Ther Technol 2012;4:25.

17. Thomas JL, Davis BC. Three-wire fixation technique for displaced fifth metatarsal base fractures. J Foot Ankle Surg 2011;50:776–9.

Current Concepts and Techniques in Foot and Ankle Surgery

Hallux Valgus Correction Using Combined Reverdin-Laird and Opening Base Wedge Procedures
A Radiographic Analysis

Lester Dennis, DPM, Jason Snyder, DPM, Tahir Khan, DPM*

KEYWORDS

- Opening base wedge • Reverdin-laird • Hallux valgus • 1st Intermetatarsal angle
- Surgery

KEY POINTS

- 1st Metatarsal opening base wedge osteotomy combined with a Reverdin-Laird procedure provides significant improvement in patients with hallux valgus deformity.
- Radiographic evaluation revealed average corrections of 1st intermetatarsal angle (IMA) of 11.875°, proximal articular set angle (PASA) of 4°, hallux abductus angle (HAA) of 18.25°, and tibial sesamoid position (TSP) of 1.75.

INTRODUCTION

The term, *hallux valgus (HV)*, was introduced by Carl Heuter[1] in 1871 to describe static subluxation of the 1st metatarsal phalangeal joint with medial deviation of the 1st metatarsal and lateral deviation of the 1st proximal phalanx. Piggott[2] reported in 1960 that 57% of patients recalled onset of HV during their adolescent years and only 3% of patients recalled HV occurring initially after age 20. Coughlin and Thompson[3] reported, in a retrospective study of more than 800 cases of HV patients who underwent correction, that the average age at time of surgery was 60. Coughlin and Thompson[3] also estimate that more than 200,000 HV corrections are performed in the United States each year.

The purpose of this study was to assess the amount of radiographic correction when a 1st metatarsal opening base wedge and Reverdin-Laird procedures are

Conflicts of Interest/Funding: None.
Level of Evidence: Level IV Retrospective.
Division of Podiatric Surgery, Department of Surgery, Wyckoff Heights Medical Center, 374 Stockholm Street, Brooklyn, NY 11237, USA
* Corresponding author.
E-mail address: tahir.khan.dpm@gmail.com

Clin Podiatr Med Surg 30 (2013) 445–450
http://dx.doi.org/10.1016/j.cpm.2013.04.010
0891-8422/13/$ – see front matter © 2013 Elsevier Inc. All rights reserved.

used in combination to treat HV. All patients in this study had a moderate to severe HV deformity, and radiographic parameters included the 1st IMA, PASA, distal articular set angle (DASA), HAA, hallux abductus interphalangeus angle (HAIA), tangential angle to the 2nd axis (TASA), and TSP (**Fig. 1**).

RESEARCH DESIGN AND METHODS

The authors conducted a retrospective study in which radiographs of 7 patients (8 total feet; 1 patient underwent bilateral correction) with symptomatic HV deformity were evaluated and radiographic measurements were taken. All radiographic measurements were taken by one of the authors (JS) using standard angle measurement techniques, as described by Coughlin and Mann.[4] Notable exceptions are that the term, *PASA*, has replaced proximal metatarsal articular angle and *DASA* is substituted for distal metatarsal articular angle. All patients had an initial presentation between 2008 and 2010 with an increased 1st IMA and were evaluated by the senior author (LD).

Inclusion criteria for this study were symptomatic HV deformity with 1st IMA greater than or equal to 12°, fully closed growth plates in the foot, and failed conservative care for at least 6 months before surgery. Exclusion criteria consisted of no previous surgical correction of the 1st or 2nd rays (metatarsal and toes) of the foot; inadequate bone stock; no other procedures performed at the same time as HV correction effecting 1st or 2nd rays; and patients with neuromuscular diseases, rheumatoid arthritis, peripheral nerve disease, or overt predisposing conditions to surgical failure.

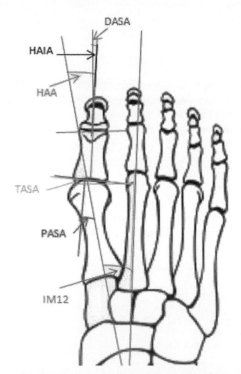

Fig. 1. Radiographic angles depicted on foot model used for this study. IM12, 1st intermetatarsal angle.

All radiographs were made in the dorsal-plantar (DP) projection with the patients standing in weight-bearing position with 1 foot on the radiographic cassette. The radiographic tube was angled 15° to vertical and was 3 m from the radiographic cassette. The center of the radiographic beam was centered on the navicular bone. The radiographs were taken with the standard 60 kV and 2 mA for DP projection of the foot. All radiographs were taken by the senior author (LD), whereas all radiographic measurements were performed by another author (JS). The authors only used DP radiographic views for their study because all the angles measured could be easily evaluated on the DP views.

SURGICAL PROCEDURE

All patients underwent surgical correction of the HV deformity by using the combined procedures under monitored anesthesia care. The surgical dissection was performed over the 1st metatarsal using a dorsomedial incision. An oblique osteotomy with the lateral cortex intact was made on the medial aspect of the 1st metatarsal perpendicular to the weight-bearing surface, using a sagittal saw 1.5 cm from the most proximal aspect of the bone. Care was taken to not violate the lateral cortex of the 1st metatarsal. A 3-osteotome technique was then used to open the osteotomy site to allow placement of internal fixation. The osteotomy splitter was then placed in the 1st metatarsal cut to determine the desired amount of correction of the HV deformity. A low profile open base wedge plate of appropriate size was then placed in the osteotomy and fixated with screws. The 2nd most proximal screw was placed across the osteotomy site. The remaining void, if any, was then filled with bone graft. Attention was then directed to the distal aspect of the 1st metatarsal, where a Reverdin-Laird procedure was performed. A sesamoid-sparing plantar osteotomy was made and an adjoining 45° cut was made just proximal to the articular cartilage of the 1st metatarsal head. The metatarsal head was then displaced laterally to approximately one-third the width of the 1st metatarsal. A single screw was then placed of appropriate length from proximal dorsal medial to distal plantar lateral direction and across the osteotomy site. The medial eminence of the 1st metatarsal was then removed with osteotomes, sagittal saw, and/or burrs, and the surgical wound was then closed in layers in the standard fashion (**Fig. 2**).

RESULTS

Weight bearing to heel was allowed with a surgical shoe and assistance devices immediately postoperatively. Initial postoperative visit was at 1 week with the primary surgeon and patients were allowed to function in a normal shoe gear at 1 month. Postoperative radiographs were taken at 1-month follow-up. All radiographs were taken by the senior author (LD) and these 1-month follow-up radiographs were used for the final radiographic measurements. After evaluating the preoperative and postoperative radiographs, the mean preoperative 1st IMA was 16.375° whereas the mean postoperative 1st IMA was 4.5°. This represents an overall correction of 11.875°, which can be attributed solely to the opening base wedge procedure using plate and screw fixation. The mean preoperative PASA was 9.25° and the postoperative value was 5.25°, which represents an average of 4° of change. Mean HAA preoperatively was 27.75° and postoperatively was 9.5° for an average change of 18.25°. Preoperative TSP was 4.25 and postoperative TSP was 2.5, with an average reduction of 1.75. Changes in PASA, HAA, and TSP are attributed to the combined opening base wedge and Reverdin-Laird procedures. TASA increased by 0.625°

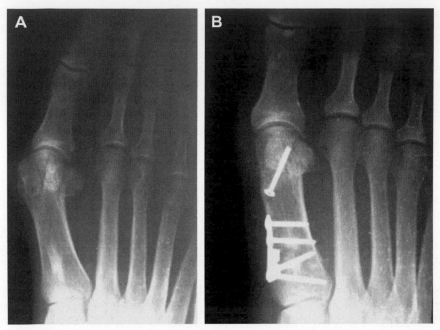

Fig. 2. Preoperative radiograph demonstrating a HV deformity (*A*) followed by surgical correction of a combined Reverdin-Laird and opening base wedge osteotomy procedures (*B*).

and HAIA increased by 2.875°, respectively. Lastly, DASA represented an average reduction of 1° (**Table 1**).

DISCUSSION

The 1st metatarsal opening base wedge procedure was initially presented by Trethowan[5] in 1923. The procedure has been scrutinized due to the inherent lack of stability of the osteotomy,[6] potential lengthening of the 1st metatarsal, HV, and decreased stability at the osteotomy site.[7] With the advanced technology in internal fixation and designs for base wedge osteotomies, however, the procedure has again become a choice in the podiatric surgeon's armamentarium. The internal fixation plates used in this study were composed of titanium with a 0.5-mm thickness.[8] The plate spacers range from 2 mm to 7 mm in 0.5-mm increments, with each 1 mm of displacement correcting 3° of the 1st IMA. The titanium screws are 2.3 mm in diameter with a length ranging from 10 mm to 30 mm in 1-mm increments.[8] The screws are fully threaded, self-tapping cortical design.[8] The thread hole drill bit is 1.7 mm.[8]

The authors' 1-year postoperative results (no radiographs were taken at 1-year postoperative follow-up visit) indicate that all the patients are completely satisfied with the cosmetic results and relate no pain or any other complaints, with the exception of 1 patient who had mild recurrence of the HV deformity. The authors think this recurrence could be due to not evaluating metatarsus primus elevatus properly during the preoperative evaluation and that this patient may have benefited from a more aggressive procedure, such as a Lapidus combined with Reverdin-Laird. Further studies are warranted to investigate different combinations of procedures, including the possibility of using a base wedge and Lapidus procedure to correct large 1st IMAs while maintaining metatarsal length.

Table 1								
Preoperative and postoperative radiographic parameters used for the study								
Patient		1st IMA	PASA	DASA	HAA	TASA	HAIA	TSP
1	Pre	18	14	8	38	4	12	4
	Post	4	12	2	20	14	12	3
2	Pre	22	14	2	24	10	4	5
	Post	6	6	2	2	4	10	3
3	Pre	12	6	2	22	2	10	3
	Post	1	2	2	4	2	16	1
4	Pre	18	6	4	30	10	1	4
	Post	3	2	4	4	10	6	3
5	Pre	16	6	4	36	8	10	4
	Post	2	4	2	8	8	10	3
6	Pre	12	6	0	20	4	10	4
	Post	8	6	2	18	2	4	3
7 R	Pre	15	6	4	20	4	8	5
	Post	4	4	4	10	4	10	2
7 L	Pre	18	16	6	32	1	4	5
	Post	8	6	4	10	4	14	2
Average change		11.875	4	1	18.25	−0.625	−2.875	1.75

Abbreviations: L, left; Pre, preoperative; Post, postoperative; R, right.

Several limitations to the study include the small sample size and the increase in the *hallux interphalangeus angle* (HIA) and TASA values despite correction of other angles. A possible explanation for the increase in HIA could be the lengthening of the 1st ray (metatarsal and toe) from the opening base wedge procedure, resulting in the extensor and/or flexor hallucis longus tendon causing a lateral pull on the distal phalanx, resulting in higher HIA. The TASA may have increased due to a medial wedge removal during the Reverdin-Laird procedure. The authors tried to minimize any errors in taking radiographs and radiographic measurements—all the radiographs were taken by the senior author (LD) and all the radiographic measurements were taken by another author (JS). The radiographic measurements of angles were performed 3 separate times by JS to further minimize any potential errors. There is, however, a possibility of error in foot placement on radiographic cassettes or amount of weight bearing on plain radiographs. The study also involves only 1-year of postoperative follow-up without postoperative radiographic measurements at that visit although long-term follow-up of several years would be ideal to determine if there is any recurrence or loss of corrections.

Other studies have looked at combined procedures for HV correction. Pochatko and colleagues[9] published on distal chevron osteotomy with lateral release, with results showing an average 5° of 1st IMA correction and 13.5° of HAA correction. Bostan and colleagues[10] studied radiographic correction in proximal crescentic osteotomy with distal soft tissue release of adductor hallucis, lateral joint capsule, and transverse intermetatarsal ligament. Preoperative measurements revealed HAA approximately 31.1°, 1st IMA approximately 15.3°, and DASA approximately 17.8°. Postoperative angles were HAA approximately 12.9°, 1st IMA approximately 8.0°, and DASA approximately 12°.

After comparing preoperative and postoperative radiographs, the authors think that their retrospective study shows that a combined opening base wedge osteotomy with a Reverdin-Laird procedure can be used to significantly reduce the 1st IMA, PASA, TSP, and HAA. The 1st metatarsal opening base wedge also allows for correction of severe angular deformities when presented with a short metatarsal length. In conclusion, these combined procedures may be considered in patients with a symptomatic HV deformity with an initial 1st IMA of at least 12° and an increase in either PASA or HAA and TSP.

REFERENCES

1. Hueter C. Klinik der Gelenkkrankheiten mit Einschluss der Orthopadie. Deutshland, Vogel; 1871 [in German].
2. Piggott H. The nature history of hallux valgus in adolescence and early adult life. J Bone Joint Surg Br 1960;42:749–60.
3. Coughlin MJ, Thompson FM. The high price of high-fashion footwear. Instr Course Lect 1995;44:371–7.
4. Coughlin MJ, Mann RA, Saltzman CL. Surgery of the Foot and Ankle. 2007. p. 207–18.
5. Trethowan J. Hallux valgus. A System of Surgery. 1923;1046–9.
6. Zembsch A, Trnka HJ, Ritschl P. Correction of hallux valgus: metatarsal osteotomy versus excision arthroplasty. Clin Orthop 2000;376:183–94.
7. Watson T, Shurnas P. The proximal opening wedge osteotomy for the correction of hallux valgus deformity. Tech in Foot and Ankle Surg 2008;7(1):17–24.
8. Available at: www.arthrex.com. Accessed September 15, 2012.
9. Pochatko DJ, Schlehr FJ, Murphey MD, et al. Distal chevron osteotomy with lateral release for treatment of hallux valgus deformity. Foot Ankle Int 1994; 15(9):457–61.
10. Bostan B, Gunes T, Erdem M, et al. Comparison of modified Lindgren-Turan operation and proximal crescentic osteotomy combined with distal soft tissue procedure in the treatment of hallux valgus. Joint Dis Rel Surg 2008;19(2):61–5.

Index

Note: Page numbers of article titles are in **boldface** type.

Clin Podiatr Med Surg 30 (2013) 451–459
http://dx.doi.org/10.1016/S0891-8422(13)00063-3
0891-8422/13/$ – see front matter © 2013 Elsevier Inc. All rights reserved.

podiatric.theclinics.com

Moving?

Make sure your subscription moves with you!

To notify us of your new address, find your **Clinics Account Number** (located on your mailing label above your name), and contact customer service at:

Email: journalscustomerservice-usa@elsevier.com

800-654-2452 (subscribers in the U.S. & Canada)
314-447-8871 (subscribers outside of the U.S. & Canada)

Fax number: 314-447-8029

Elsevier Health Sciences Division
Subscription Customer Service
3251 Riverport Lane
Maryland Heights, MO 63043

*To ensure uninterrupted delivery of your subscription, please notify us at least 4 weeks in advance of move.

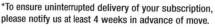
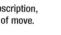

Printed and bound by CPI Group (UK) Ltd, Croydon, CR0 4YY

21/10/2024

01777130-0001